P9-DDR-956

M. E. Anderson
2/6/93

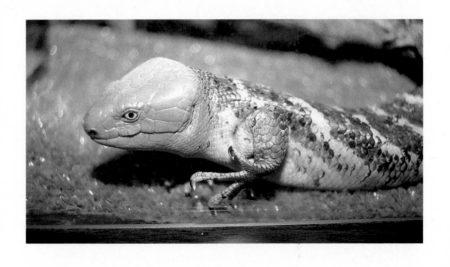

REPTILE DISEASES
KW-197

CONTENTS

Preface 4
Getting a Reptile 6
Care of Reptiles 16
Some Reptilian Anatomy 30
Disease Recognition and Treatment 38
Infectious Diseases 52
Parasitic Diseases 70
Environmental Diseases 86
Some Reptilian Psychology 106
Medication for Sick Reptiles 116
Suggested Reading...126
Index...127

Photographers: William B. Allen Jr., Dr. Herbert R. Axelrod, Horst Bielfeld, Dr. Warren Burgess, Guido Dingerkus, John Dommers, E. Elkan, Isabelle Francais, Michael Gilroy, Rolf Hackbarth, B. Kahl, S. Kochetov, Ken Lucas (Steinhart Aquarium), K.T. Nemuras, Louis Porras, Elaine Radford, Harald Schultz, R.S. Simmons, E. Zimmermann.

Title page: A male wood turtle (*Clemmys insculpta*).

Originally published in German by Franckh'sche Verlagshandlung under the title *Krankheiten der Reptilien*. First edition 1985 by Franckh'sche Verlagshandlung. ©Copyright 1990 by T.F.H. Publications, Inc., for English translation. A considerable amount of new material has been added to the literal German-English translation, including but not limited to additional photographs. Copyright is also claimed for this new material.

© Copyright 1990 by T.F.H. Publications, Inc.

Distributed in the UNITED STATES by T.F.H. Publications, Inc., One T.F.H. Plaza, Neptune City, NJ 07753; in CANADA to the Pet Trade by H & L Pet Supplies Inc., 27 Kingston Crescent, Kitchener, Ontario N2B 2T6; Rolf C. Hagen Ltd., 3225 Sartelon Street, Montreal 382 Quebec; in CANADA to the Book Trade by Macmillan of Canada (A Division of Canada Publishing Corporation), 164 Commander Boulevard, Agincourt, Ontario M1S 3C7; in ENGLAND by T.F.H. Publications Limited, Cliveden House/Priors Way/Bray, Maidenhead, Berkshire SL6 2HP, England; in AUSTRALIA AND THE SOUTH PACIFIC by T.F.H. (Australia) Pty. Ltd., Box 149, Brookvale 2100 N.S.W., Australia; in NEW ZEALAND by Ross Haines & Son, Ltd., 82 D Elizabeth Knox Place, Panmure, Auckland, New Zealand; in the PHILIPPINES by Bio-Research, 5 Lippay Street, San Lorenzo Village, Makati Rizal; in SOUTH AFRICA by Multipet Pty. Ltd., Box 235 New Germany, South Africa 3620. Published by T.F.H. Publications, Inc. Manufactured in the United States of America by T.F.H. Publications, Inc.

REPTILE DISEASES

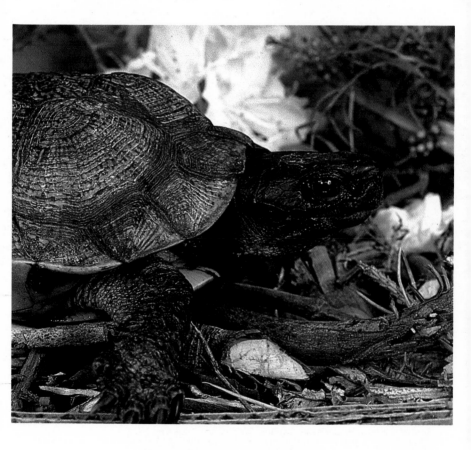

BY ROLF HACKBARTH
Translated by U. Erich Friese

Preface

Keeping reptiles has become increasingly popular in recent years. This trend is indeed gratifying, provided, of course, that it is based on the genuine desire to learn more about these animals. Regrettably, reptiles are all too often treated with bias and prejudice. It is necessary to understand these animals better so that they can be protected, which in turn stops them from becoming endangered. Less commendable, of course, is the only too common desire merely to have an exotic and unusual hobby.

Due to widespread global habitat destruction, many reptiles are already threatened with extinction. Most of these species are now strictly protected and/or subject to more or less stringent trade restrictions. Therefore, it is of paramount importance that those species that are still commercially available are not only protected but also—if possible—bred in captivity. Prerequisite for this is an adequate knowledge that facilitates species-correct housing, proper care, and early recognition and specific treatment of diseases.

There are many books on reptile keeping; however, popular books on the diseases of reptiles are less common. This book is a contribution toward closing this gap and providing help and support to hobbyists faced with particular reptile disease problems. Our current knowledge about the diseases of turtles, snakes, and lizards of course cannot make any claims of completeness, yet research in this sector has made great advances during the last decade. Many losses now can be avoided and numerous diseases now can be effectively treated.

I would like to take this opportunity to express my sincere thanks to Dr. Raethel and Dr. and Mrs. Gerber, as well as to many others for their contributions in the areas of parasitology, mycology, and pathology. My particular appreciation goes out to the late Prof. Mertens, who early on encouraged me to persevere—in spite of frequent setbacks—and to continue on with my work in the relatively little-known areas of research and treatment of reptile diseases.

Rolf Hackbarth

Opposite: A common tegu (Tupinambis teguixin), *also known as the black or banded tegu. Tegus are considered difficult to keep, but once acclimatized they can live up to ten years in captivity.*

4

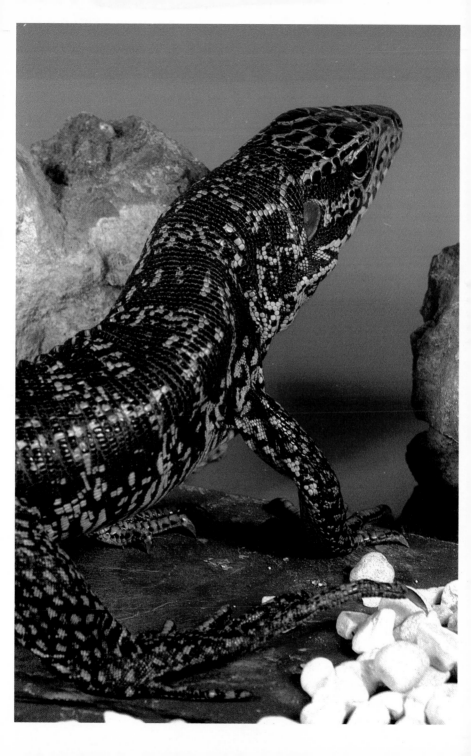

Getting a Reptile

Getting and keeping a reptile must be a carefully thought-out decision in order to avoid, as far as possible, unpleasant surprises.

For instance, all family members must be consulted beforehand, as should landlords and other individuals who may also become involved, to ascertain whether there are any objections to keeping reptiles—especially snakes. Nothing is more unpleasant and often legally difficult for the owner of a newly bought animal—and for the animal itself—than to have to return the animal to the vendor.

Before a decision is made to get a particular type or species, it is imperative to learn as much as possible about this animal. This can be done by researching the relevant literature and questioning experienced reptile hobbyists about particular requirements. How much space is needed (not only for a juvenile specimen, but also for adults)? What is the required food and how much is eaten? Is it possible to provide an optimum, varied diet throughout the year? Is it a solitary animal or can it be kept together with other animals? Which other species are

*Corn snake (*Elaphe guttata*). Before acquiring a reptile or any other pet, be sure all family members—and landlords—give their consent.*

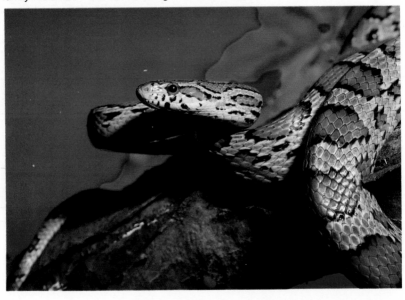

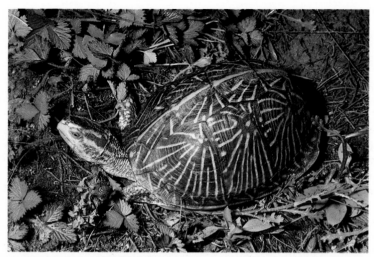

*The eastern box turtle (*Terrapene carolina bauri*) is highly variable in form— rarely are two specimens the same.*

compatible? How must the terrarium be set up so that species-correct housing is provided?

After these questions have been answered and the terrarium has been set up accordingly, the next step can be contemplated: acquisition of the animal(s). It is strongly advisable to take a sufficiently large cotton bag and possibly a styrofoam box along to provide safe transport for the newly acquired animal(s). Styrofoam boxes are particularly well suited since they can be heated up and will actually retain the heat for some time. If the animal has to be transported over a considerable distance—particularly during cold weather—a styrofoam box is mandatory. A hot water bottle should be placed inside so that there is an even temperature.

HOW DO YOU RECOGNIZE A HEALTHY ANIMAL?

A healthy reptile shows the following characteristics:

—clean, shiny, dry skin, without pustules, open sores, weeping wounds, or remnants of old (unshed) skin;

—well-muscled body without visible vertebra, pelvic bones, or ribs;

—tight, well-conditioned limbs with smooth claws, the skin firm at bases of limbs;

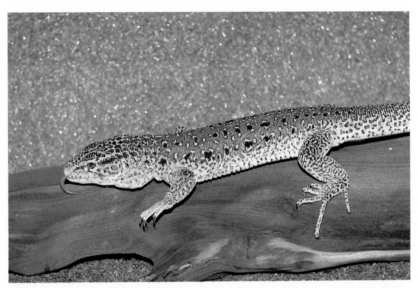

*Spotted monitor tegu (*Callopistes maculatus*). Despite the beliefs of some hobbyists, healthy and tame reptiles do flick their tongues. This action helps the animals perceive changes in their environments.*

—firm tail base;

—lips free of injuries or skin growth;

—oral mucous membranes without coating and undamaged;

—eyes and nostrils open, clean, and not encrusted;

—cloacal opening clean, closed, not encrusted with feces or mucus;

—in turtles, a rigid, evenly formed carapace without deformed or missing scutes or unusual growth forms;

—active tongue-flicking in snakes and some lizards.

The insistence by some dealers that tame reptiles do not flick their tongues is incorrect, because reptiles, particularly snakes, must flick their tongues in order to perceive and recognize their surroundings. All reptiles—even those that have adapted to humans—will actively flick their tongues as soon as there are changes in their immediate surroundings. Specimens that do not respond in this manner are not healthy.

It is advisable to have the dealer take the animal from the terrarium so it can be examined more closely. Particular attention should be paid to the abdominal scales, the skin folds along the inner region of the upper thighs and bases of the legs, the eyes, the ear openings, and any neck folds in search of ticks and mites.

The dealer should also be asked to test the specimen for its vitality and mobility. When touched, a turtle will relatively rapidly retract its head and limbs into the carapace for protection. When placed on its back, a lizard will attempt to return to its natural position with agility and speed. Exceptions are those species that as a defensive measure pretend to be dead when handled. This "rigor" will cease after a short period of time.

Sick specimens are often emaciated and show their vertebrae, pelvic bones, and ribs.

They may have loose skin (hunger folds) along the posterior abdominal region, upper thighs, and neck caused by muscle atrophy; the base of the tail appears caved-in; and the eyes are sunken deep into their sockets and are usually closed. Such a "death candidate" may open its eyes briefly, but when picked up it will invariably hang limply, moving its limbs lethargically and showing little inclination to fight or flee. Refrain from buying an animal that has an obvious cheesy coating on the oral mucous membranes or along the rows of teeth (mouth rot) or that emits continuous whistling or rattling respiratory sounds. If its eyes and nostrils are slimy or encrusted or it has small bubbles formed in front of

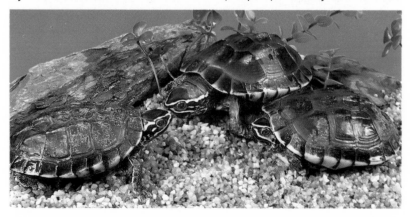

*A trio of Malayan snail-eating turtles (*Malayemys subtrijuga*). Healthy turtles will rapidly draw their heads and limbs into the shell (carapace) when they feel threatened.*

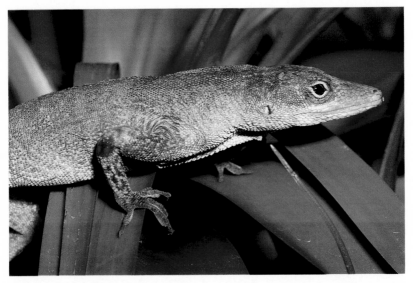

Bite wounds, like those seen on this anole, are not uncommon. Normally they will heal quickly; however, during the next molt particular attention should be paid to the scarred area to see that it is shedding properly.

the nostrils, leave it alone. If the cloaca is coated, incompletely closed, or surrounded by pink skin (rectal prolapse), or if the skin is covered by pustules, sores, or weeping wounds, don't buy it. Caution is also advised when the terrarium contains regurgitated, partially digested food or soft, foul-smelling feces. Animals in such obviously poor condition will rarely survive the renewed stress of transport and transfer into another terrarium.

From experience it can be said that absolutely flawless reptiles are rarely available. After all, there are species that will

develop minor skin lesions even when touched very lightly. Small scars, slightly scraped noses, and old, well-healed injuries should not discourage you from acquiring the animal, provided its movements are not too severely affected.

There is always a certain inherent risk involved when buying reptiles, because the feeding behavior of many species often cannot be observed for some time after the purchase (certain species can go without food for quite some time). Consequently, it may take days or even weeks before it can be determined if a specimen will feed properly.

When buying "wild-caught" specimens (reptiles collected in the wild in their natural habitat and then exported) the risks of incurring problems during the period of acclimation to captivity are, of course, substantially higher than with animals that are captive-bred. Newly imported specimens may be aggressive, resulting in injuries to the handler that can lead to serious complications if these bites are from venomous reptiles not recognized as such. These animals are already weakened and disturbed from the trauma of capture and transport. The new surroundings, captivity, and other influences may make some shy and apathetic. These "newcomers" require much patience, intensive and responsive care, careful observation, and much experience.

*Sand lizard (*Lacerta agilis*). This particular species must not be kept in surroundings that are too dry.*

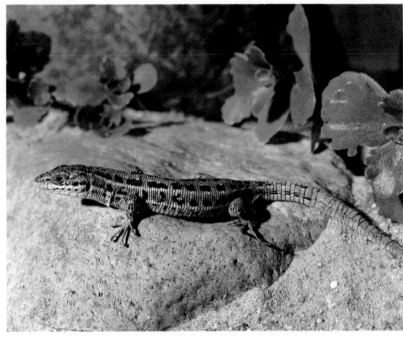

Finally, the big moment has come: you exchange cash or a check for your new acquisition—carefully wrapped in a securely tied small cotton sack—and you are about to start on your way home. Stop! Right here the first problems can occur if proper care is not taken. If a suitable styrofoam box is not available you have to make sure that the cotton sack and its contents—protected against cold, drafts, and excessive heat—are transported home as quickly as possible. If you travel by car, make sure that nothing heavy is placed on top of the cotton sack

*Aesculapian snake (*Elaphe longissima*). Note the broken and fused scales on the head; these were probably caused by an injury early in the animal's life.*

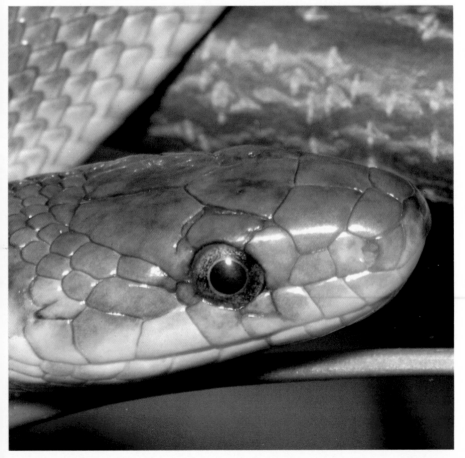

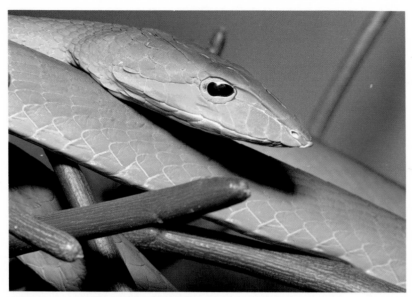

Asian long-nosed tree snake (Ahaetulla prasina). *This species is not easy to acclimatize, since it feeds mainly on lizards.*

or can accidentally fall on it. While these words of warning may sound unnecessary, accidents like this happen all too often!

After arriving home it is advisable that the new arrivals are not immediately placed into the newly set up terrarium. Instead, all new animals should be kept initially in a quarantine terrarium for about four to eight weeks to observe and monitor them for possible diseases. This procedure is always applicable when the newly acquired animal is an addition to others of the same species already in the terrarium, or if the new arrival is an imported specimen.

Before an animal is released into quarantine, it should be bathed in warm water (about 30°C, 86°F). Since newly arrived animals are often reluctant to go into the water, the bathing dish must be covered by a screened or otherwise perforated lid and weighted down with a rock. The water level must be adjusted so that the animal can easily raise its head above water. For small lizards and snakes it is advisable to place a rough-edged piece of wood in the dish to give the animal something to hold on to or climb up on to get its head above water.

THE QUARANTINE TERRARIUM

A quarantine terrarium must be uncluttered and almost sterile—it must be easy to clean and disinfect. Best suited are nearly square containers made of glass or plastic. Although plastic containers are cheaper, they tend to become stained (clear acrylic becomes "cloudy") from frequent applications of disinfectants, and eventually they start to look less appealing.

The bottom of the quarantine container should be covered with newspaper, which is very absorbent and can easily be changed.

Heat should be provided by means of a heating coil or heating pad inserted between two thin sheets of pressboard that are covered with plastic or sheet metal. The cable leading out of the terrarium is neatly tucked into one of the upright corners and well protected by a cover strip of wood or metal. A small radiant heater or infra-red source attached to the lid of the terrarium also can be used. The spartan decoration of a quarantine terrarium should include a wood or cardboard box ("hide box") under which the animal can withdraw if need be. A drinking dish and possibly also a suitably large bathing bowl complete the quarantine setup.

Below: Example of a quarantine cage. This fiberglass model has a sliding front panel that provides easy access to the inside. **Opposite:** Profile of an adult leopard gecko (Eublepharis macularius).

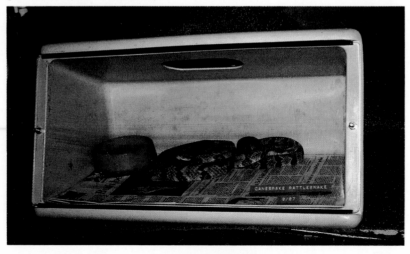

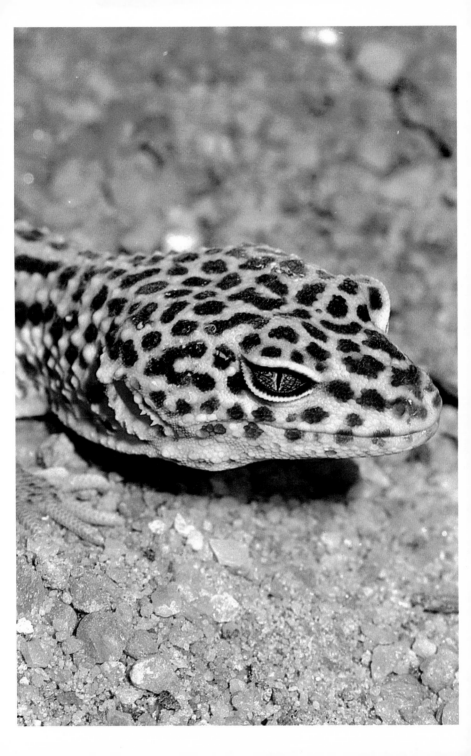

Care of Reptiles

Attentive care, species-correct housing, a varied diet, and painstaking cleanliness are of paramount importance for the health of captive reptiles.

SPECIES-CORRECT HOUSING

Proper (species-correct) housing requires adequate knowledge of the natural habitat and mode of life of the newly acquired animal. Large animals and those that are very active require a terrarium with a large open area. Climbing species should be given a relatively high terrarium. Aquatic species need a proper bathing facility. Those that prefer a dry habitat should be given a terrarium with a sand substrate for burrowing and possibly also a rocky basking area. Species that occur in a highly varied habitat in nature should be afforded a choice between patches of dry and damp substrate, some warmer and some cooler areas, and open space as well as hiding places. On the other hand, arboreal forms, those living in trees and bushes, should have lots of plant material in the terrarium so that branches and leaves can provide adequate cover for comfortable resting and sleeping places.

DIET

The first mistake in reptile keeping—and one that may ultimately lead to the death of the animals—is often made in feeding the animals. One common vice among reptile hobbyists is to give far too much food, so that diseases that do not normally occur in a particular species in the wild are virtually provoked. Any hobbyist must realize and appreciate the difficulties normally encountered by reptiles in nature while hunting their food. Let us take a gecko, for instance, that attempts to capture an insect in the wild. Quite often the intended prey either flies or jumps away before the gecko can get to it. How often does a python miss the desired mammal or bird that it urgently needs to satisfy its feeding urge? How long does a turtle have to wait until a fish swims past close enough to be swallowed? Obviously there is a reason why some reptiles can undergo more extreme fasting periods than any other vertebrates. Particularly, snakes are known to be able to fast for often prolonged periods of time, where six months or more without having to feed are not uncommon.

In a terrarium situation food animals can not run or fly away, and consequently reptiles tend

*Opposite: A pair of red-eared sliders (*Pseudemys scripta elegans*). This species grows quickly; therefore, space may become a problem for the keeper.*

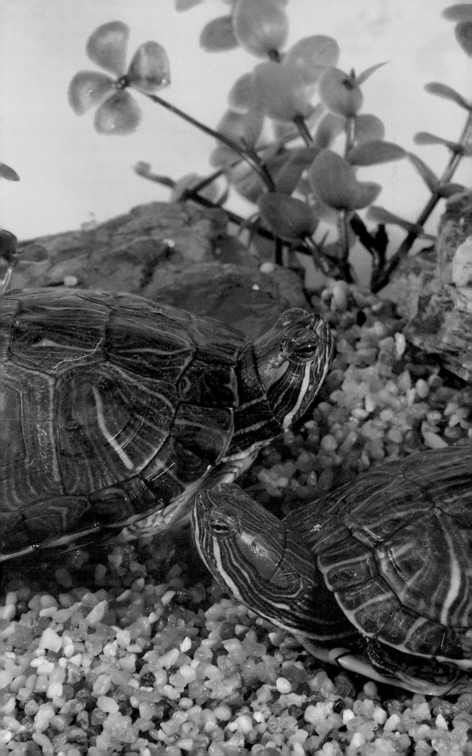

to get too fat very quickly. Therefore, a responsible reptile hobbyist has his charges occasionally undergo a "fasting period," which does not have to occur at regular intervals. During these periods food is not given at all, so the animals have to draw on their own body reserves. Moreover, using this method can help bridge those periods when food is indeed scarce and hard to come by (i.e., during the winter months). However, such fasting periods only make sense when the normal diet is sufficiently varied. Under these conditions the keeper can easily go on vacation for three to four weeks with a clear conscience, knowing that the reptiles will not starve to death. The author has been practicing this method for years and has always found his reptiles to be in the best of health upon his return. However, it is imperative that there is always sufficient water available, especially for those species that must have frequent or constant access to it.

The question now is: where do we get a sufficiently varied diet, and what does "varied" actually mean for particular species?

Apart from so-called food specialists, such as horned lizards (*Phrynosoma*) that feed mainly on ants or snakes that

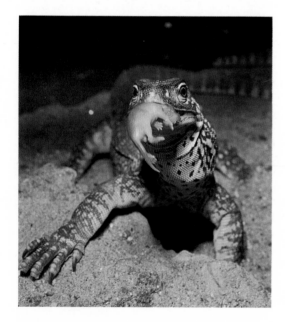

*Reptiles that feed on small mammals, birds, and bird eggs should occasionally be given this type of food in captivity. This Gould's monitor (*Varanus gouldi*) is eagerly feeding on a newborn mouse or "pinkie."*

*Maintaining food specialists in captivity requires considerable effort to provide the proper diet. Some species are sufficiently adaptable and can adjust to food that is similar in nutritional value. The pink-tongued skink (*Tiliqua gerrardi*), however, continues to prefer snails.*

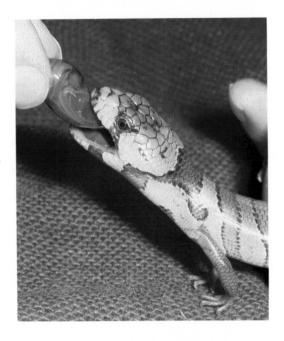

prey mainly on lizards (animals such as these should be kept only by experienced hobbyists!), the pet shop should be able to provide some, if not all, of the dietary items needed for most commonly kept reptiles. Nevertheless, it is advisable to check with the dealer as to what he has available in the line of suitable food at the time the reptile is purchased. It is also important to know whether the dealer anticipates any seasonal variations in the availability of particular food items. There are dealers who sometimes specialize in reptile food species (mice, crickets, mealworms) and then have these available throughout the year. If there is sufficient space in the basement or somewhere else in a house and if there is enough spare time available, the hobbyist may well wish to breed some of the *main* food species himself. There is deliberate emphasis here on the word "main." It is virtually impossible to breed all organisms that make up the normal diet of one or possibly even several different reptile species. Such a breeding program would require considerable space and too much care and effort.

Now we come to another

major point: If the diet of a particular reptile species consists, for instance, mainly of plant material (herbivorous species), this does not mean that only well washed and dried lettuce leaves would be sufficient. Quite to the contrary; the range of suitable dietary items for such herbivorous species includes at least dandelions, clover, sorrel, tomatoes, slices of cucumber, strawberries, bananas, apples, and other fruits. There should also be some insects, small mammals (rodents), and pieces of raw lean meat (all according to the size of the species) available for herbivorous reptiles. The same applies to reptiles that are primarily carnivorous (meat-eaters)—a diet consisting exclusively of mice and mealworms is equally unsuitable. During the warmer months of the year such a one-sided diet can easily be supplemented with earthworms, caterpillars, spiders, meadow plankton (small insects and spiders caught in a sweep net), etc., all available free-of-charge from the wild. However, when meadow plankton is used it is important to check first whether this comes from meadows that have been sprayed recently with chemicals. Specifically, you should avoid areas directly under fruit trees that are sprayed with insecticides and fungicides,

Below: some hobbyists breed food animals, such as crickets, in order to supplement the diet of their reptilian charges. *Opposite:* A young Coachwhip (Masticophis flagellum). Members of this genus are nervous and very active.

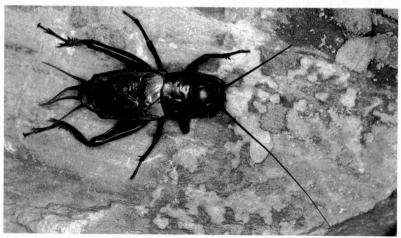

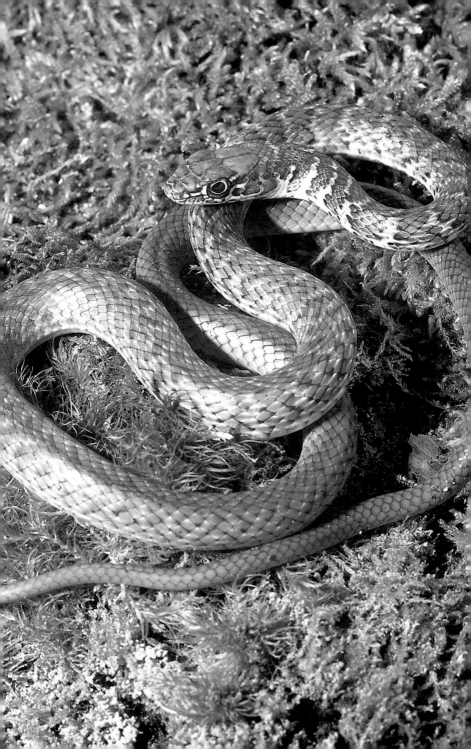

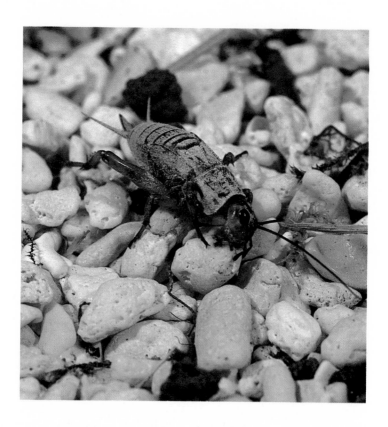

substances that commonly leach onto the grass below and then to its insect residents! For similar reasons, fresh green leaves should not be picked from alongside roads! Many carnivorous reptiles also like the occasional piece of vegetable and sweet fruit. It is best to try out a number of food items in order to determine the preference patterns for individual animals.

Reptiles should be fed at a time when they are most active, which then gives a good

Before feeding wild-caught insects or greens to your reptiles, be sure they have never been sprayed with pesticides of any kind.

indication of what is actually eaten and what food is rejected. Moreover, live foods such as meadow plankton, mealworms, waxmoths, and other small arthropods and even small mice are then not able to hide and

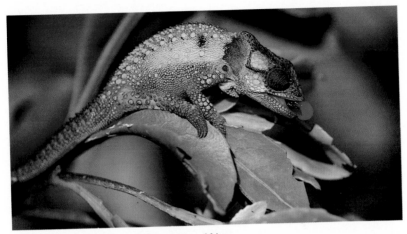

A chameleon photographed in its native Africa.

escape being eaten. For even better control, food can be offered individually by hand using feeding forceps. Greens, fruits, and vegetables should be cut into small pieces and offered in stable feeding dishes—after all, we humans also dislike sandy bananas or strawberries!

Left-over food, especially when alive, must never be permitted to remain in the terrarium

Adult chameleons eat houseflies, while their young subsist on aphids and fruitflies.

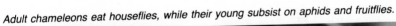

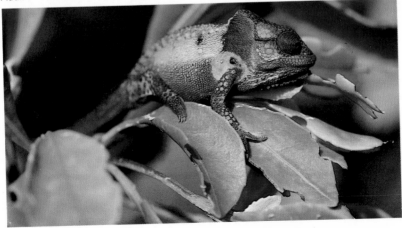

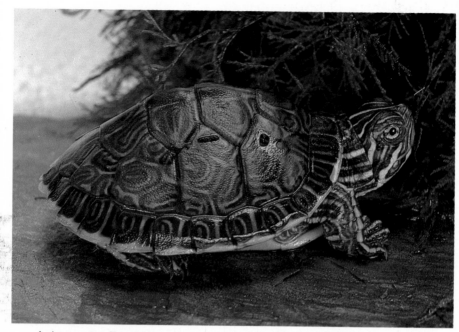

*A river cooter (*Pseudemys concinna hieroglyphica*). If you plan to let your reptile have free run in a particular room, remove all plants, as many are toxic.*

uncontrolled. This is particularly important with rodents. It has happened that sometimes the hunted has become the hunter! Rodents have a tendency, particularly at night, to gnaw on unsuspecting resting reptiles, causing serious bite wounds or even death. Although this may sound like a horror story, it nevertheless happens all too often, so it must be mentioned here.

DRINKING AND BATHING FACILITIES

Just as important as a varied, species-correct diet is the supply of drinking water and the provision of suitable water containers for bathing.

The size and depth of such water containers depend on the size of the reptiles to be served and their drinking and bathing requirements. The containers preferably should be made of glass or ceramic, since these materials are easily cleaned and—most importantly—can be disinfected without being affected by the disinfectants.

Drinking containers should be placed in such a way that they are not polluted by debris from the terrarium substrate (sand, gravel, etc.). It is advisable to place them in a corner where they can be secured with a few large rocks. Drinking containers should be relatively shallow, since most reptiles take up liquid through licking. For tree-dwelling reptiles it is sufficient to spray the leaves frequently, since most species like to lick water off wet leaves or catch water drops falling from the leaves.

The bathing dish should never be higher than the height of the animal that is to use it. In order to make it easier for the animal to get out of the water, a few small stones should be placed on the bottom of the dish. It is imperative that both drinking water and bathing containers be cleaned thoroughly and refilled with fresh water every day.

CLEANLINESS—THE FIRST COMMANDMENT!

Out of consideration for the animal there should be no need to stress the point of regular cleaning of the terrarium and related components—after all, we too generally do not like to live in dirt and filth! But we have the choice to stay or leave, unlike

Some turtles need a large area in the terrarium for bathing. Before purchasing such an animal, be sure you can provide for it properly.

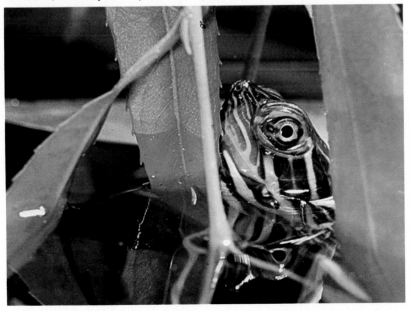

reptiles in captivity that can not leave the terrarium. More specifically, painstaking cleanliness is imperative as a protective measure against disease outbreaks and transmission. Feces and decaying left-over food are often sources for various disease germs, so these will have to be removed from the terrarium as quickly as possible. Useful

every use! Never use the same tool in two or more terrariums without first disinfecting it!

Sudden and abrupt movements should be avoided when removing debris from a terrarium! Some reptiles become nervous at the slightest disturbance and will readily crash their heads into the terrarium walls. Therefore, use only slow and deliberate

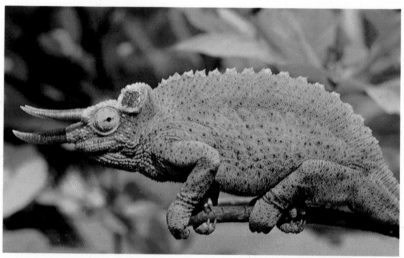

Three-horned chameleon (Chamaeleo jacksoni). All items, including branches and rocks, must be removed from the terrarium and cleaned or replaced regularly.

implements for their removal are long, strong stainless steel forceps, angled shovels with long handles, discarded soup spoons, etc. These tools have to be properly disinfected after

movements and always keep an eye on the animal(s)—there is no need for bites caused by disturbed animals. Gloves that extend all the way up to the elbows are often very useful for working around newly acquired or aggressive animals.

In spite of meticulous efforts to remove all debris, some will always remain on the ground and stuck to branches, terrarium walls, and decorations inside the terrarium. For that reason the entire terrarium should be dismantled at regular intervals and all components should then be meticulously cleaned and disinfected.

Before embarking on such a major cleaning operation, all animals have to be removed and temporarily housed elsewhere. Cotton bags are ideally suited for that purpose: the animals can be accommodated individually and injuries are avoided. Moreover, the bags are small and handy and can be easily transported. However, bags with animals

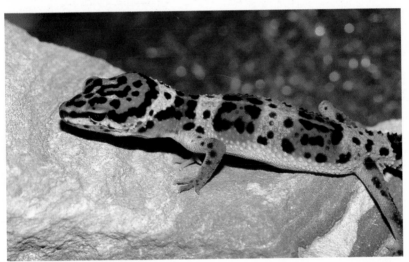

A young leopard gecko (Eublepharis macularius) lounging on a rock. If a terrarium rock seems difficult to clean, replace it when you dismantle the tank for maintenance.

disinfected. The substrate and hard to clean branches and rocks should be completely replaced; everything else from inside the terrarium and, of course, the terrarium itself must be scrubbed thoroughly and then inside must not be left lying around carelessly; although they provide a certain amount of protection, they do not keep out drafts and cold, and they provide no resistance to pressure (as from being stepped on).

Therefore, it is advisable to place the bags with their reptilian contents into a sufficiently large plastic dish that is then deposited in a suitably warm location (*never*, of course, in direct sun).

Be careful when removing the substrate. You may be one of those lucky hobbyists who discover eggs laid by their charges! Great care must be exercised when transferring such eggs. Most experts suggest that their position not be changed (i.e., not turned or placed upside down). It may be possible to leave them where they are and place a sufficiently large container over the entire clutch, including a section of the substrate. This protects the eggs against damage while the terrarium is cleaned (but be very careful if using disinfectants) and prevents terrarium inmates from feeding on the eggs or newly hatched young. Unless a screen cover is used, be sure to lift the cover every day or so (very carefully!) to check for hatching.

Once the terrarium has been emptied completely (or at least as far as possible) it is treated with a commercially available disinfectant, throughly washed out, and then dried. When using a disinfectant it is very important to follow the manufacturer's instructions for use (details

*Egg of a hog-nosed snake (*Heterodon sp.*) beginning to hatch. If you are lucky enough to find eggs in your reptile tank, be careful—try to leave them where they are if at all possible.*

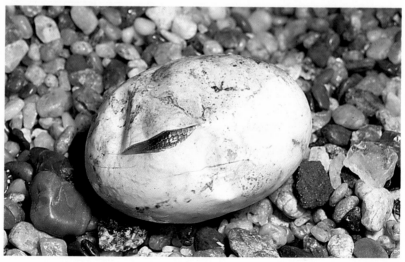

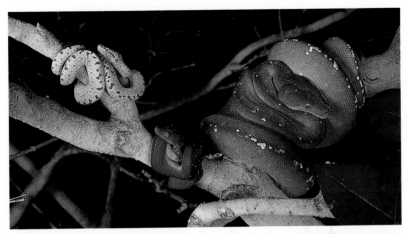

A green tree python (Chondropython viridis) *with two of its young. As you can see, juveniles of this species range in color from yellow through orange and brown to red.*

about concentration levels, etc.). It appears superfluous to mention that such chemicals must be kept away from children and animals!

It also goes without saying that all electrical appliances, such as the heater, radiant heat source, and lighting, must be disconnected.

All items from inside the terrarium must be thoroughly brushed, disinfected, rinsed off, and then dried.

Before the terrarium is set up again and the reptiles re-introduced, it must be permitted to air out, preferably overnight. Should this advice not be adhered to, it is possible that, due to residual disinfectant vapors, poisoning can occur

among the animals. Poisoning symptoms can take the form of apathy, a wide open mouth—sometimes to the point of vomiting—and cramps. Problems also can occur if the animals are re-introduced into an under-cooled terrarium, so the terrarium must be slightly warmed up before the animals are returned.

In order not to upset the animals unduly and to give them an opportunity to re-acclimate to clean and new-smelling surroundings, the bags are opened cautiously and are slowly turned inside out in the terrarium. This permits the animals to find their own way out of the bag at their own pace.

Some Reptilian Anatomy

Reptiles are cold-blooded (poikilothermic), usually egg-laying vertebrates, that are—on the basis of body shape—divided into three basic groups:

1) lizard-like, with (usually) five-toed, clawed limbs;

2) snake-like, without limbs;

3) turtle-like, with a compact body enclosed in a bony carapace.

The lizard-like reptiles include the true lizards, the crocodilians, and the tuatara. The snake-like reptiles include the true snakes, quite a few lizards with reduced or no legs, and the usually legless amphisbaenids, a group of uncertain relationship. Turtles are of course just turtles.

All reptiles have a dry, tough skin with few glands; there usually is a multilayered horny cover in the form of variously developed scales or shields. Since this horny cover does not grow to keep pace with increasing body size, it must be shed periodically (molted). It is shed either in the form of individual pieces (most lizards), in its entirety (snakes), or in the form of individual plates on the carapace (turtles). Most reptiles lay eggs encased in calcareous or parchment-like shells. They are fertilized internally with the aid of unpaired or paired male copulatory organs and are deposited via the cloaca, a mutual opening for the excretory and sex products.

The form of the internal organs is dependent upon body shape of the respective animals and therefore in nearly all reptiles, except in turtles, is more elongated than broad and flat. Reptiles have a heart with a double atrium, but there is an incompletely divided ventricle, so that arterial blood and venous blood mix in the heart. The red blood cells (erythrocytes) are oval and have a nucleus (mammalian red blood cells are rounded and do not have a nucleus).

Reptiles are lung-breathers. Their lungs are simple, internally strongly furrowed, elongated sacs of light red coloration. In snakes the left lung is reduced or completely absent, and in some lizards both lungs are not of equal size. A diaphragm, which separates the chest cavity from the abdominal cavity, is not present in reptiles.

The elongated liver contains a pigment (melanin) that gives this organ, when in healthy condition, a black-dotted or black-striped appearance. The kidneys are usually flat, lobate, elongated structures located near or behind elongated supra-renal bodies.

Opposite: *A pair of collared lizards (Crotaphytus collaris) male and female. The male is the larger, stouter animal.*

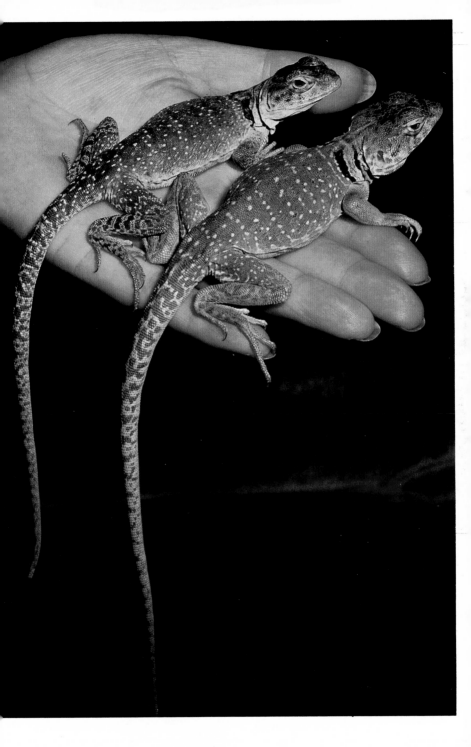

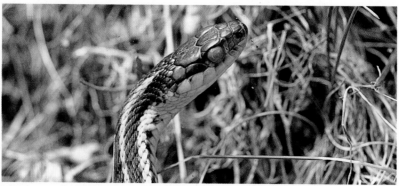

*Note the cloudy blue eye on this common garter snake (*Thamnophis sirtalis*), a sure sign that it is about to molt.*

Male (testes) and female (ovaries) sex organs are almost always paired. In male reptiles there is a copulatory organ (penis) that is pushed out from the cloaca. In lizards and snakes the penis is a paired structure, the hemipenes. Excess fat is accumulated as fatty tissue in the abdominal cavity.

SNAKES (SERPENTES)

There are more than 3000 snake species; most are concentrated in the tropics and subtropics, where they occupy

A discarded snake skin. The skin of a newly molted snake is much brighter than the old one.

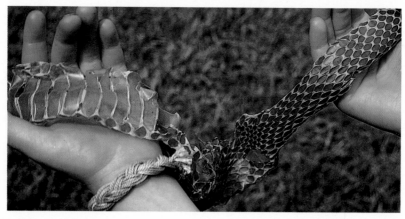

greatly diversified habitats.

Snakes are elongated, limbless, scaled reptiles. Their skeleton consists of a skull, made up of bones that are substantially movable relative to each other, and a variable number of vertebrae. All vertebrae are equipped with ribs, except the anterior neck vertebrae and the tail vertebrae. A shoulder girdle is absent in all species, but the pelvic girdle is still present in primitive groups.

extendable. Consequently, even small snakes can swallow relatively large prey. The pointed teeth are bent backward so that prey once grasped can no longer break loose, but instead becomes more deeply enmeshed in the teeth. Snake eyes are distinctive because of their "staring look" due to a transparent "window" developed from the fused eyelids, which protects the eye from dirt and debris. This window (the brille or

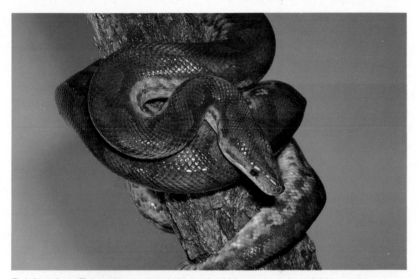

*Rainbow boa (*Epicrates cenchria*). Note the iridescent scales of this species.*

Eye and nose cavities are located laterally on the skull. The jaws and the roof of the palate are connected by ligaments so that the mouth is enormously

spectacle) is replaced during each molt. Cloudy eyes may indicate an imminent start of the next molt.

The tongue is long and forked

and serves primarily as an olfactory (smelling) organ. During the familiar tongue-flicking the tip of the tongue picks up aromatic substances from the air and transfers them to a special organ (Jacobson's organ) located in the roof of the oral cavity, which then actually perceives the aromatic substances.

Due to the elongated body shape, the internal organs of snakes are correspondingly elongated and are arranged in a longitudinal direction. The esophagus and stomach are highly distensible. The lungs are always uneven in size; usually the right lobe is elongated and the left one has often totally regressed.

Males possess a paired copulatory organ (hemipenis).

Females usually lay large parchment-shelled, elongate-oval eggs that can usually be left unattended. Some snakes are ovoviviparous, the already fully developed young breaking out of the thin egg membrane while still inside the female or minutes after the shell-less eggs have been laid.

LIZARDS (SAURIA)

Most of the about 3000 or so lizard species live in the tropics and subtropics, where they occupy diverse habitats: they can be ground-dwellers or live as burrowers in the soil; they can have an arboreal mode of life, living in trees and shrubs; some species are found under stones, on rocks, along river and lake banks, and even in the sea (Galapagos iguanas). The body

Common Madagascar day gecko (Phelsuma madagascariensis). Phelsuma *geckos are arboreal—they spend a good deal of time in trees.*

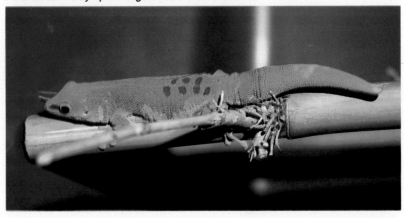

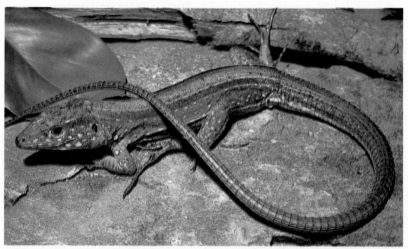

Dotted racerunner (Cnemidophorus lemniscatus). Racerunners dwell on the ground and require spacious terrariums.

shape of lizards can assume all sorts of transitional forms, from well-developed four-legged species with five toes to legless, snake-like forms. The legs are always lateral, pointing away from the trunk, resulting in a close to the ground, crawling type of locomotion. Some species are capable of dropping their tail when endangered (autotomy) and so confuse the attacker.

The skeleton consists of the skull and a usually long vertebral column with two limb girdles and the legs. The tail can be long and slender or short and thick. The skull bones are firmly attached to each other and possess only marginal mobility. Eye sockets and nostrils are located laterally on the head. The eyes are usually equipped with movable lids, but in some species these have become fused in snake-like fashion into a transparent window or "spectacle." Many species also possess a third rudimentary eyespot (parietal eye) on top of the head; its function is not yet fully understood, but it is not capable of actual vision.

The body of a lizard is covered with smooth, rough, spiny, or keeled scales. The scales may have bony cores in some armored species.

Males are equipped with a paired copulatory organ (hemipenis). Females are predominantly egg-laying; only a relatively few species give birth to live young. The eggs are usually covered by a parchment-like shell and are deposited at protected sites, where they are left unattended. Only a few species provide actual brood care.

*Red-eared slider (*Pseudemys scripta elegans*). Turtles have good eyesight and sense of smell, but their hearing is not well developed.*

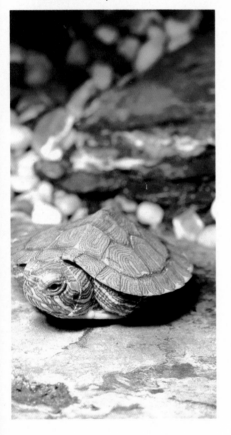

TURTLES (TESTUDINES)

The distribution of the approximately 220 turtles species includes all warm regions on earth. One can distinguish among land, marine, and freshwater (aquatic) turtles, depending upon their habitat.

Turtles have a compact body that is enclosed in a carapace consisting of a dorsal section and an abdominal section (plastron). The carapace, from which only the head, the four legs, and the tail protrude, is covered by either a leather-like skin or horny plates. The skeleton consists of the skull, eight neck vertebrae, ten trunk vertebrae, two sacral vertebrae, and a variable number of caudal (tail) vertebrae. The ribs are fused with dermal cartilages to form the dorsal carapace. The eye sockets are located laterally (occasionally dorsally) along the side of the head, with the nostrils up front. The jaws are toothless but are equipped with strong horny covers. Depending upon the method used for hiding the head inside the carapace in case of danger, one distinguishes between neck retractors and neck benders: the neck retractors (cryptodires) pull in their head so that it is retracted in a vertical S-shaped bend. On the other hand, neck benders (pleurodires) place their head horizontally in an S-shaped curve between the upper and lower

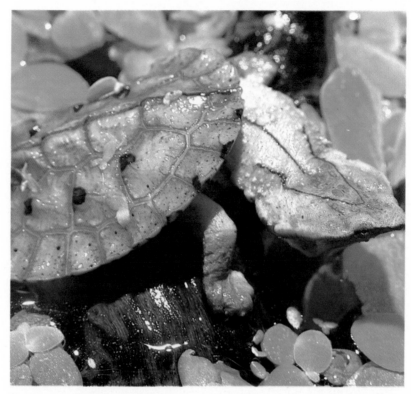

The matamata (Chelus fimbriatus) lives in slow-moving or still jungle waters. It grows to a large size but does not require a great deal of space, as some other species do.

anterior edges of the carapace; thus they are known as side-necks.

Turtles can see very well and react extremely fast in response to vibration stimuli. Their sense of smell is quite well developed, but their hearing is less acute. Due to the compact body structure, the internal organs are placed close together.

The males have only a single copulatory organ (the penis). All turtles are egg-layers. The eggs are spherical or elongated and are enclosed by a calcareous or parchment-like shell. The females usually dig a pit into which the eggs are deposited and then cover them with soil. Thereafter, the clutch is left unattended.

Disease Recognition and Treatment

In spite of the old proverb that an ounce of prevention is better than a pound of cure, reptiles in captivity tend to get sick despite species-correct housing, optimum care, and a varied diet. Regrettably, there are—at times—diseases that can be fatal. The sooner a disease is recognized and identified, the sooner proper corrective treatment can be initiated; the sooner proper medication is administered, the greater are the chances of full recovery.

EARLY RECOGNITION OF DISEASES

Any hobbyist who knows his animals and who observes them closely will quickly detect the first signs of a disease, simply because reptiles—just like any other living animal—reflect physical or physiological problems and subclinical (hidden) diseases by changes in their normal behavior. However, this behavior can vary quite substantially from species to species and even among the members of the same species. Such behavioral changes can manifest themselves in apathy, asthenia (lack of physical energy), and reluctance to feed, as well as in aggression, biting, and nervous pacing in the enclosure. For instance, reptiles with an inflammatory bacterial disease in the lower abdomen can become extremely aggressive and attempt to bite at the slightest touch. Yet animals with parasitic intestinal diseases tend toward a reluctance to feed, increased fluid intake, and apathy (listlessness). An infestation with ectoparasites (mites and ticks) or skin abscesses (accumulation of purulent material) usually provokes rubbing, scratching, and scraping along rough objects (rocks, stones, etc.) by the affected animals. Moreover, parasitic infestations often cause the animals to remain in their bathing containers for extended periods of time. A slightly open or wide open mouth can be indicative of diseases affecting the mouth, pharynx, air passages, or lungs. Encrusted nostrils, eyes, and mouth are often symptomatic of colds. Dragging limbs or refusal to use particular limbs (indicated by prolonged resting or reluctance to move particular limbs) can be a sign of fractures or dislocations (luxations).

Such observations, particularly when supplemented by changes in the appearance of particular animals, will often convey a

*Opposite: Male double-crested basilisk (*Basiliscus plumifrons*). This animal's crest is diseased or has worn away with age.*

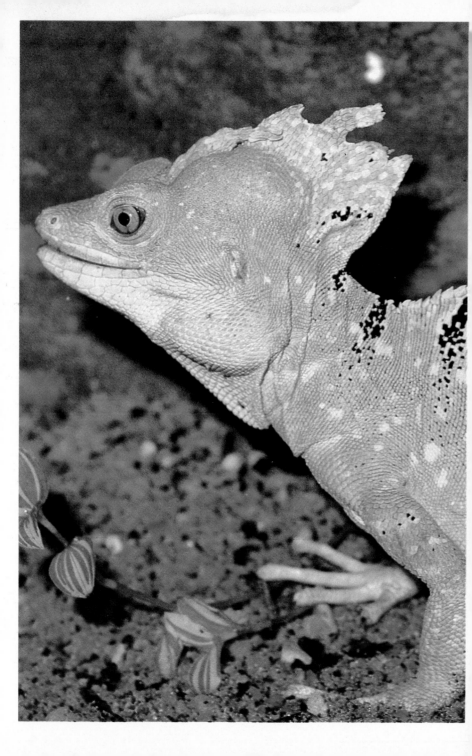

rather clear picture of a developing or already established disease. Particularly the skin and eyes can be valuable indicators of the state of health of a reptile. A healthy specimen has a shiny, smooth, and dry skin. However, an animal in poor condition will have a matte and dull skin where the colors have faded, sometimes to a point where the animal appears unicolored. Scales are often spread (raised) because of a loss of condition and weight, giving the animal an appearance of "untidiness"; these conditions are often further compounded by considerable molting (skin shedding) difficulties. The normally clear, shiny eyes become dull and lose their gloss (not to be confused with the milky clouding up of the eyes just prior to molting).

Folded skin along the abdomen due to emaciation or caved-in muscle sections along the legs and at the base of the tail indicate a severe and advanced stage of a disease. Regurgitation of partially digested food or soft and slimy feces (caused by diseases of the digestive tract, but possibly due to poisoning from food treated with insecticides) require immediate treatment.

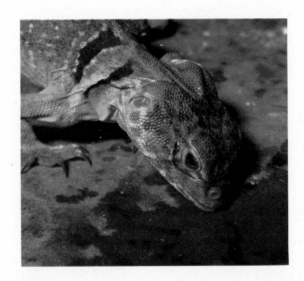

*When a reptile takes frequent and prolonged drinks, it is a sure sign that it is ill. The collared lizard (*Crotaphytus collaris)*, for instance, drinks only moderately when healthy.*

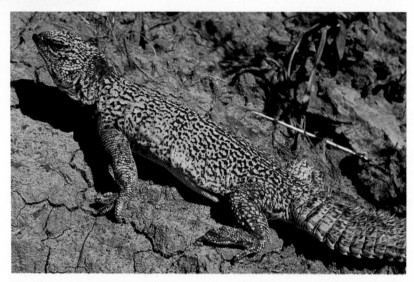

The African spiny-tailed agamid (Uromastyx acanthinurus) and other spiny hard-tailed lizards often have trouble molting, with remnants of skin remaining until the next molt. Lukewarm baths will help soften the pieces of old skin so they can be cautiously removed.

On the other hand, refusing to feed does not always indicate a health problem. Instead, this is often a sign that stronger, more aggressively feeding siblings prevent another animal from feeding. Alternatively, a change in diet may be indicated. However, when there is a persistent refusal to feed, even if all other animals are removed from the enclosure and the diet has been sufficiently varied, a disease problem should be

A green, or Carolina, anole (Anolis carolinensis) during the molt.

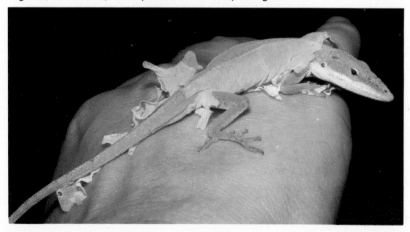

suspected. It should be remembered that reptiles have "psyche," and they can react adversely to a change in surroundings or to the death of a partner, often with a reduced desire to feed.

If an animal displays distinct behavioral changes it has to be examined closely. Are there any changes on or inside the mouth? What does the cloacal region look like? Are the muscle sections, especially along the

deposited, wet feces can be used for this purpose. A piece the size of a cherry is removed and placed inside an air-tight unbreakable container (plastic vial, refrigerator container, or tightly sealed plastic bag). This is sent out to the nearest test laboratory or simply taken to a cooperative veterinarian.

Animals that show symptoms of a fracture or dislocation should be x-rayed by a veterinarian.

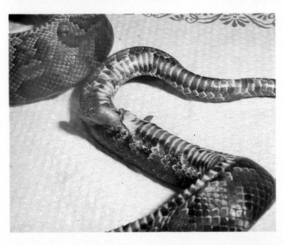

This snake was injured in the cloacal region during capture or transport. Since the open wound was not treated immediately, the subsequent inflammation spread to other areas. An intensive antibiotic treatment induced complete healing of the affected area.

legs and at the base of the tail, still taut and in good condition? Is there any change in consistency or color of the feces?

In order not to miss anything it is imperative that a microscopic examination be made of the feces to check for parasites, especially worms and worm eggs. Only fresh, newly

HOUSING AND CARE OF SICK REPTILES

Trying to catch a reptile in a well-decorated terrarium, particularly when it has lots of hiding places, is not an easy thing at the best of times. Can you imagine what it would take to handle and medicate a sick animal once or twice a day? Therefore, it is strongly

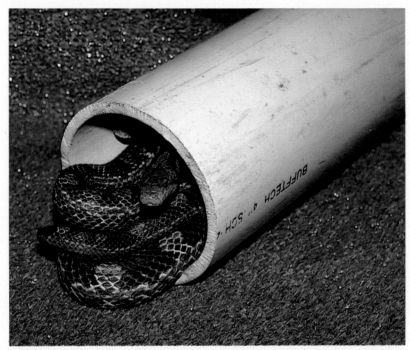

A PVC pipe is useful for removing a snake from its quarters without handling it directly. When the snake crawls into the pipe, the pipe can simply be lifted out of the cage.

recommended that you isolate such animals in a quarantine or isolation terrarium for closer observation and better treatment, also preventing other animals from becoming infected. This type of container has the advantage that, due to its spartan interior, it is easy to clean and the animal can be monitored more closely. At the same time, newly deposited feces are promptly found and removed for a rapid test.

For most reptiles, the temperature in the quarantine container during the day should not exceed 30°C (86°F) and must not drop below 22°C (72°F) at night. The humidity must be between 40 and 60%.

Aggressive animals are best placed inside a tightly woven linen or cotton sack. This sack is draped over one hand (covered if necessary by a heavy-duty welder's glove) that is then used to grab the sick animal behind the head. The sack then is pulled over the animal's entire body. When the sack is closed it is important to make sure that none of the extremities have gotten caught. The sack is then

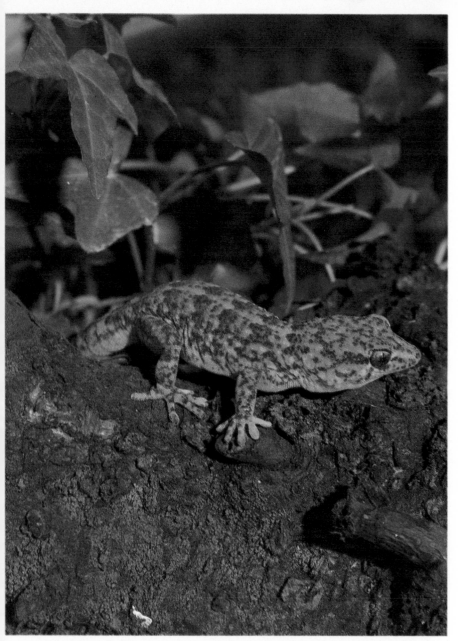
Wall gecko (Tarentola delalandi). A terrarium arrangement such as this is not suitable for quarantine. Quarantine terrariums should contain only the bare necessities.

tied off with a string or tie wire. For treatment purposes—once again—the head is grabbed with a glove-covered hand inside the sack and the remainder of the animal's body is uncovered.

Experience has shown that placing such animals in sacks has many advantages. Applied dressings are not dislocated or even slipped off. Ointments and lotions will adhere to the inside of the sack and are therefore in constant contact with the animal's body and the affected areas. Also, ectoparasites that have dropped off the sick animal can be spotted quickly and easily removed. These sacks are also easy to clean and disinfect. The reptiles are quickly caught and can be easily treated. Moreover, the administration of medication is without problems when the animal's body is well-protected inside the sack with only the head protruding; this protects the keeper against sharp claws and painful lashes from the tail.

Sacks with reptiles inside should be placed close to an adequate heat source and in a well-ventilated location without drafts. Plastic pans are useful for that purpose. The sick animal must have regular access to drinking water. Even if the animal is at first unwilling to drink from a bowl held in front of it, it will adapt after a while to such an arrangement.

While the diseased animal is being held in isolation, the regular terrarium is cleaned out thoroughly and disinfected so a possible infectious disease is not transferred to other occupants of the terrarium or possibly even right back to the same animal when it is returned.

ADMINISTERING MEDICATION

Administering medications to reptiles can often be a rather trying experience. In reptiles that feed at regular intervals this does not represent a problem: these animals can receive the medication—as long as it can be given orally—in their food. However, animals that do not feed at regular intervals or those that completely refuse to feed require much patience and great diligence.

It is advisable that sick animals be placed in a cotton sack with their head restrained. With the other hand (protected by a heavy-duty leather glove) the mouth is cautiously opened and the animal is firmly grabbed behind the head. A pencil is then delicately forced between the jaws (caution—not too much pressure on the head!). The administration of liquid medication or tablets dissolved in water requires the use of a one-way syringe that is extended with a section of soft plastic tubing. The tube is slowly and very cautiously inserted down the esophagus so that none of the liquid enters the air passage, forcing the liquid slowly down the esophagus. Afterward the head is held high for a while and the outside of the throat is gently massaged so that all the liquid is actually swallowed.

Before any medication is administered to a sick animal the following recommendations should be adhered to. In order to consult a veterinarian. It can happen that certain medications, when administered at the same time, may cause complications. Cloacal applications and intramuscular injections should (intravenous injections *must*) be administered by a veterinarian—he or she is trained and experienced in this and therefore knows best how and exactly where such injections are done. For this purpose a sack is very

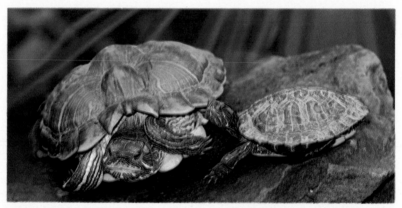

Above: *A pair of red-eared sliders* (Pseudemys scripta elegans). *If you suspect any animal of illness, quarantine it immediately.* **Opposite:** *One important sign of good health is clear, bright eyes like those on this iguana.*

achieve a quick and optimal cure, it is advisable to expose the sick animal(s) to an elevated environmental temperature. This causes increased metabolic activity that facilitates a more rapid absorption and distribution of the medication. Before several medications are administered simultaneously you should useful, too, because even veterinarians do not like to be exposed to and distracted by claws, tail lashes, or strong bites, especially since reptiles rarely ever appear as patients in a veterinary clinic.

If for some reason you have to administer intramuscular (i.m.) or intraperitoneal (i.p.) injections

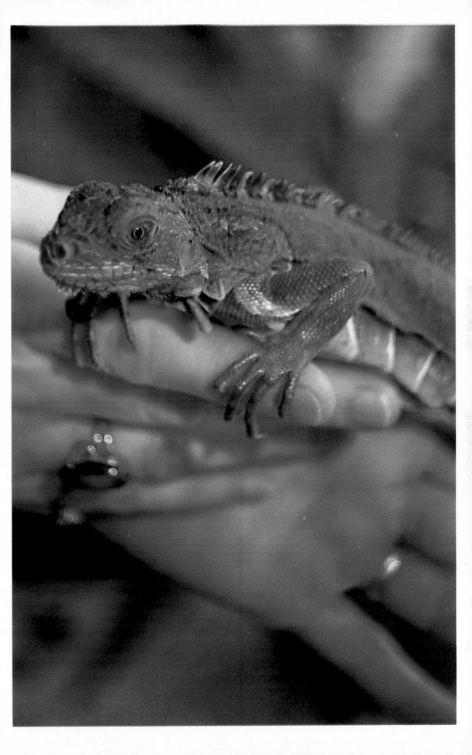

yourself, the following recommendations should be observed. Small reptiles should never be injected with more than 0.5 ml (medium size animals maximum 2 ml) intramuscularly. A larger volume does not disperse well in the thin musculature and would possibly form large-area hematomas that disappear very slowly. If small reptiles have to be injected with a large volume, this should be done i.p. (intraperitoneally) into the lower abdominal cavity, but never more than 0.5 ml at a time. Use narrow-gauge hypodermic needles, otherwise medication could be lost through oozing out of the injection canal and the

dosage would become inaccurate. Inject the medication slowly and evenly in order to assure a better distribution and prevent any return flow (oozing).

Intramuscular (i.m.) injections are usually administered into the upper thigh musculature or the strong tail musculature; subcutaneous (under the skin) injections (s.c.) are best given into the abdominal wall since it is strongly vascularized.

Surgical procedures (operations) must be done only by veterinarians. The hobbyist is strongly advised against trying his or her own hand at this!

Simple wound dressings can of course be applied and

African rock python (Python sebae) undergoing tick removal. Minor treatments such as removal of external parasites can often be done at home.

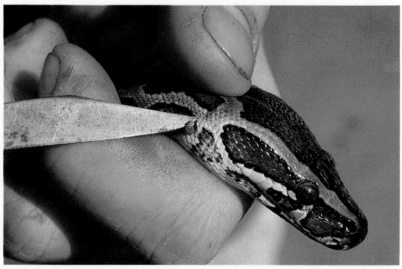

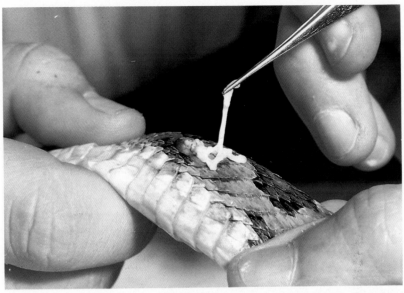

A wound being treated by a vet. Complicated treatments and/or operations must not be performed by anyone but a qualified veterinarian.

changed by anyone. Here the first commandment is painstaking cleanliness. Since dressings with poor adhesive properties will not adhere properly to rough, scaly reptilian skin (and moreover are often ripped off by the animals), it is recommended that the entire dressing be covered with wide surgical adhesive tape much beyond the edges of the actual dressing. Unfortunately, this means that the wound is sealed off virtually air-tight, so such a solid dressing *must* be changed daily. The wound should be aired (under observation) for a while

so that the weeping areas dry up faster and heal better.

Once the wound is closed and dry, a dressing is no longer required and ointments, powders, etc., can be applied without dressing. It is advisable to apply ointments, etc., in a thicker layer and for a longer period of time, since the reptilian skin is rather tough and absorbs the active ingredients very slowly. In addition, much of the ointment is wiped off from the wounds without dressing during the normal movements of the animal. Medications in powder form adhere poorly or virtually not at all, and it is advisable to rely mainly on salves, ointments, and pastes.

AUTOPSY

It does, of course, happen that in spite of all care and attention a terrarium animal sometimes dies. If there are no obvious external causes for such a death, that animal should be autopsied

advancement in the identification and treatment of reptile diseases in general.

Dead specimens sometimes can be examined by knowledgeable vets, by vets on the staffs of some zoos, and by specialists at appropriate colleges or veterinary hospitals. Your local veterinarian or perhaps a local zoo may be able

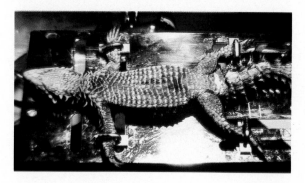

A lizard carcass undergoing autopsy. This animal was infested with ticks, which led to skin damage, secondary bacterial infections, death of tissue (necrotisation), circulatory collapse, edemas in the lung— and death.

in order to determine the exact cause of death. This should be done in any event so that a possibly infectious disease can be brought under control early and the other animals in the same terrarium can be given preventive medication. An autopsy is also needed so that possible mistakes in maintenance and nutrition can be avoided in the future. All relevant details should be recorded. The compilation of statistics on reptilian diseases and mortalities represents substantial scientific

to give you more detailed information.

Here are some guidelines for sending animal carcasses. The dead animal should be sent out as quickly as possible, because dehydration and/or partial decomposition makes an accurate diagnosis very difficult or even impossible. In addition, frozen specimens may not be diagnosed accurately (histology is virtually impossible from frozen tissues). The dead animal should be placed in a tightly sealed plastic bag and stored in a refrigerator (and preferably be

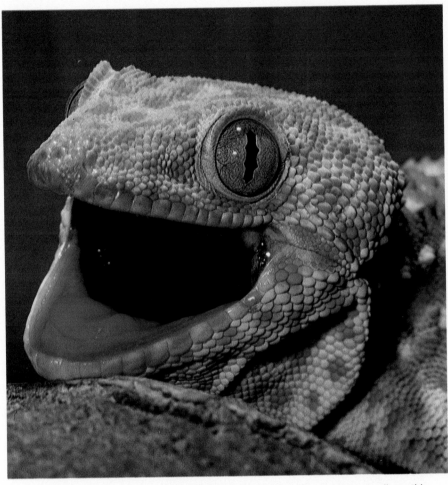

A brightly colored Tokay gecko (Gekko gecko). Note the complex pupil on this animal.

sent out for autopsy the same day). For the actual shipment the animal (inside its plastic bag) is packed in a styrofoam box, which should also contain a second plastic bag with ice cubes to provide refrigeration. The shipment must contain an accompanying letter outlining all available data on the animal (approximate age, sex as far as is known, size, length of time in captivity, its diet, behavior, and any unusual changes).

Remember that mail delivery will not accept leaking parcels, so be sure everything is *tightly* sealed.

Infectious Diseases

VIRAL INFECTIONS

A virus is the smallest disease-causing pathogen. One of its characteristic features is its ability to cause cell division in host cells, but it is unable to reproduce itself outside the host's cells. Unfortunately, little is know about infectious viral diseases in reptiles. Viral infections have to be considered when no other influences (e.g., bacteria, worms, burns, and injuries) can be shown to be involved in tumors, skin lesions and necrosis, pox-like sores, growths, swollen organs, and other organic changes.

The treatment of virus-related diseases in reptiles depends upon the overall condition of the animal involved and the severity of the disease. Affected reptiles that clearly show they have no chance of survival because they have lost too much condition and are already approaching death should be put down (euthanized) so that they do not suffer needlessly.

Virus-based swellings and tumors (if not already too large) can be removed surgically. Purulent skin necrosis and skin lesions can be cleaned out and then receive further treatment with antibiotic powder and ointments. However, such procedures should be left to the experienced veterinarian!

Minor purulent or open infected skin injuries are treated twice daily with an application of antibiotic ointment. Experience has shown that germ-free dressings contribute significantly to the healing process. They prevent subsequent invasion by other pathogens such as bacteria and fungi that would adversely affect healing.

UV or infra-red radiation treatments (minimum radiating distance 80 cm, duration 30–60 seconds, eyes must be protected in order to avoid blinding) can contribute significantly to the healing process.

BACTERIAL INFECTIONS

Bacteria are microscopically small single-celled organisms without a true cell nucleus. Depending upon their respective shape, one distinguishes cocci (spherical), bacilli (rod-shaped), spirilli (screw-shaped), and spirochaetes (elongated, spiral-shaped). Most live as saprophytes or parasites. Saprophytic species derive their nutrition from dead plant or animal tissues; among them are species that are of significance for causing fouling, decay, and fermentation. Among the parasitic forms there are

Opposite: *A healthy looking one-month-old green water dragon* (Physignathus cocincinus).

52

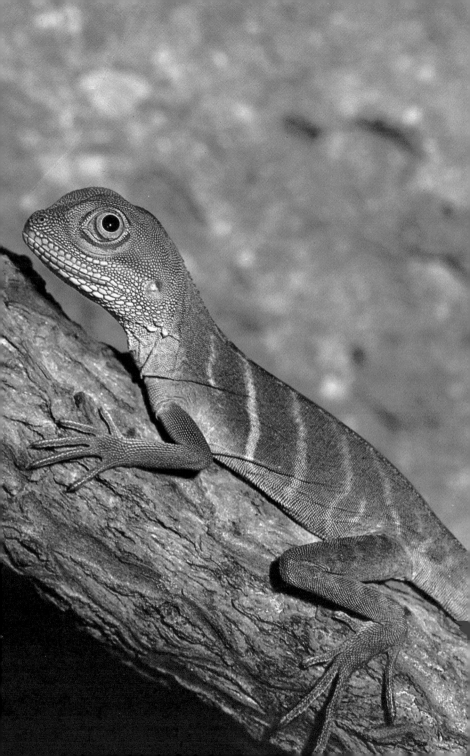

numerous species that cause dangerous diseases in plants and animals. Most bacteria require oxygen in order to live (aerobic bacteria). Some can survive without oxygen (anaerobic bacteria). Nearly all bacteria multiply by means of transverse partitioning (fission).

Regrettably, bacterial infections are not uncommon in captive reptiles. Some individual reptiles are merely carriers (hosts) and transmitters of bacteria (e.g., *Salmonella*) without themselves becoming ill. A bacterial infection in reptiles is in most cases preceded by a loss of condition due to inadequate nutrition, insufficient care, and stress due to capture and transport as well as due to injuries and other ailments. Strong and healthy specimens usually have an adequate body

defense system (sufficient antibodies) so that they generally can resist an infection. With early recognition, bacterial infections can in most cases be successfully treated and fully cured with the necessary medications (antibiotics).

Mouth Rot (stomatitis ulcerosa) The most dreaded bacterial disease in reptiles— and one that still causes substantial losses—is mouth rot (stomatitis ulcerosa). The causative agents of this disease—bacteria of the groups *Pseudomonas, Aeromonas*, and *Proteus*—accumulate in the oral mucous membrane and there cause infections, swellings, and a cheesy discharge.

Those cases of mouth rot that were identified and examined by the author were based almost

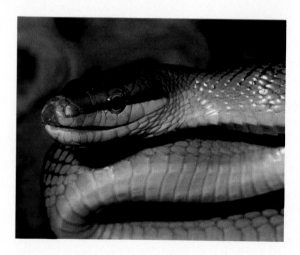

Mouth rot in reptiles can be caused by B-vitamin deficiency or through bacterial inflammation, which is often preceded by physical damage to the animal. This red-tailed rat snake (Gonyosoma oxycephala) bashed its snout; this wound should be closely monitored and treated with antibiotics to prevent mouth rot from developing.

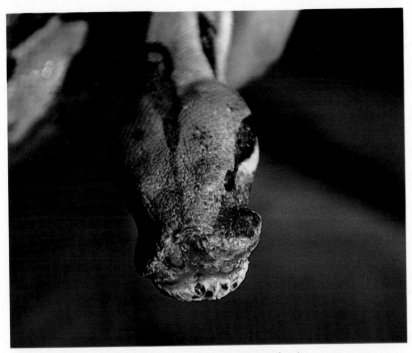

*Close-up of a boa constrictor (*Boa constrictor*) with mouth rot.*

exclusively on secondary infections caused by injuries, poor physical condition, and monotonous environmental influences. Records on subjects like nutrition, care, temperatures, etc., kept by some of those hobbyists owning the diseased animals—especially by those who had encountered repeated cases of mouth rot—indicated that the animals had been kept under conditions of excessive repetitiveness or monotony. It was exactly this background in the care and maintenance of these animals that actually facilitated the outbreak of mouth rot. The following example will clarify this point.

A particular hobbyist some time ago received three snakes in spring. The two larger ones were housed at a constant temperature in a species-correct terrarium located in the basement. The third, a small python, was placed in a terrarium located in a room on the first floor. This terrarium was essentially barren and contained only a light source. In the hobbyist's opinion this was sufficient since the room was heated (even at night) and maintained an adequate temperature. In late October the two snakes in the basement showed mouth rot, but the snake on the first floor was completely healthy and without any signs of beginning mouth rot. What had happened?

The temperature in the basement terrarium had been kept constant by thermostatically controlled central heating. The gradient (at night) was only about 2–3°C. The smaller snake encountered substantially greater temperature variations since the light was turned off at night (about 7–8°C or more). In September the weather turned colder, but since the thermostatically controlled heating system was not re-adjusted, the snakes were suddenly exposed to greater temperature variations. This led to a sort of physical weakening of the body system in the snakes (due to environmental influences) that favored the development of mouth rot. Such experiences have been encountered by the author many times.

Puff adder (Bitis arietans), a venomous snake, with mouth rot. Note the infected tissue below the fangs.

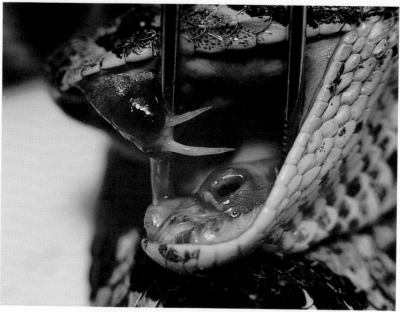

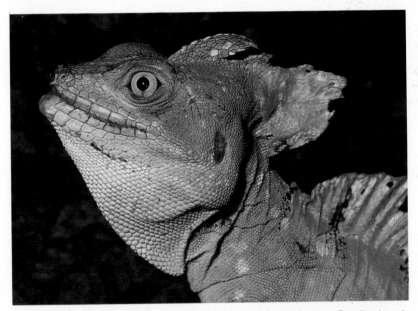

*Double-crested basilisk (*Basiliscus plumifrons*) with a bruised snout. Reptiles kept in terrariums that are too small run the risk of injuries that can lead to infection and mouth rot.*

Under natural habitat conditions reptiles do not encounter constant temperature, humidity, soil moisture, weather conditions, or food availability. Instead, these tend to vary at all times. In reptiles these ever-changing environmental factors activate physiological defense mechanisms that make the body and its organs resistant to many diseases so that an adequate immune-response level is obtained. Organisms that cannot adapt and adjust do not survive!

Mouth rot, regardless of its immediate cause, is always preceded by an infection of the oral mucous membrane (stomatitis); foam, accompanied by soft hissing, exudes from the slightly opened mouth of the affected animal. If the mouth is cautiously opened, one discovers that the mucous membranes along the inner and outer tooth rows and those at the lip margins in the lower jaw show a bright red inflammation. At this stage this disease can nearly always be treated successfully.

With the aid of a cotton swab the affected areas are touched

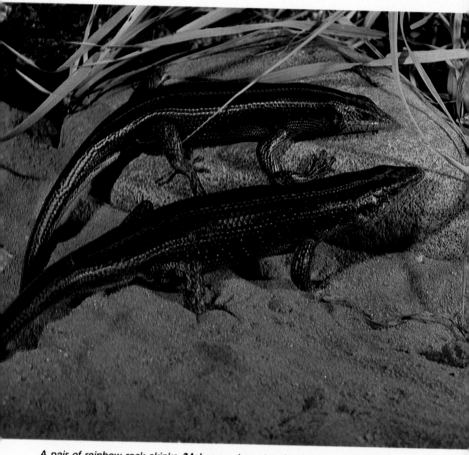

*A pair of rainbow rock skinks (*Mabuya quinquetaeniata*), also known as five-striped mabuyas.*

up several times a day with an oral disinfectant until healing has been accomplished. Oral antibiotics can also be administered as support therapy (this should be supplemented by a single dose of vitamin C).

Painting the affected areas with a 3% suspension of sulfamerazine has also proven to be effective. Early recognition of mouth rot followed by immediate treatment is important since serious diseases of the digestive tract have often been implicated as having had their origin in mouth rot.

If an inflammation of the mucous membrane is not recognized early and treated without delay it will quickly advance to actual mouth rot: upper and lower jaws are covered with pinhead-size bright red pustules with light tops,

animal and inhibit its food intake. If the diseased animal is not already too exhausted it often attempts to rid itself of the diseased tissues by rubbing and scraping the jaws along branches and rocks in the terrarium. If up to that point mouth rot has not been diagnosed, one would by then certainly be able to smell it!

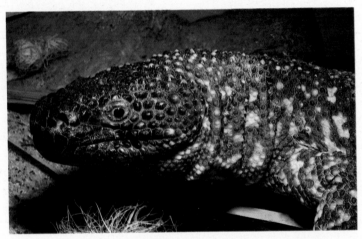

*Mexican beaded lizard (*Heloderma horridum*), a venomous species.*

mainly along the tooth rows and lip margins. The oral mucous membrane itself is pale. At an even further advanced stage the pustules become purulent and open abscesses and sores begin to form that are painful to the

During further progress of the disease the roots of the teeth and the jaw bones sustain damage and the teeth begin to fall out. Without immediate treatment at that point the animal will likely die.

In order to be able to provide quick and specific relief a veterinarian or similarly qualified individual should be contacted for an identification of the bacteria involved (based on tissue smears and culturing) and for an antibiotic sensitivity test for a rapid determination of the most effective medication.

Strictly adhere to the following procedures for the treatment of mouth rot. The purulent and necrotic layers in the mouth should be removed daily with a cotton swab, and the affected mucous membrane should be coated with a 3% sulfamerazine suspension. If possible, administer orally an antibiotic with vitamin A and C supplements. A moderately strong circulatory preparation (vasopressor) should be used as support therapy. If these medications are not swallowed or are regurgitated, they must be injected intramuscularly or intraperitoneally. It is imperative that the animal receives sufficient liquid during the entire treatment period! Instead of water a physiological saline solution should be given.

When the disease is in its early stages and the animal is still feeding, it is advisable to reduce the amount fed at each meal but increase the feeding times so that not too much energy is diverted during the digestive process but instead is used for healing and tissue regeneration. Reptiles that can fast for extended periods of time may not need to be fed at all during the treatment period. If solid food is regurgitated, a beaten egg mixed with lean chopped meat and liver and then "laced" with the medication should be given instead of solid food. Food of this consistency is usually retained and easily digested.

If, however, the stomach or intestine is affected by the disease, an oral administration or cloacal injection of sulfamerazine via a button cannula, combined with vitamin C and A supplements, has shown excellent results. Animals injected with sulfonamides have also shown good healing results, but only when combined with vitamins. Infra-red radiation, camomile baths, and the addition of sulfamethazine to the drinking water further support the therapy and facilitate good results.

The author was not able to implicate mycosis (fungal infection) as a cause of mouth rot. Fungi do occur occasionally on a secondary basis, which makes the treatment somewhat more difficult.

Opposite: A proper diet will go a long way toward keeping your reptile happy and healthy, like this green anole (Anolis carolinensis).

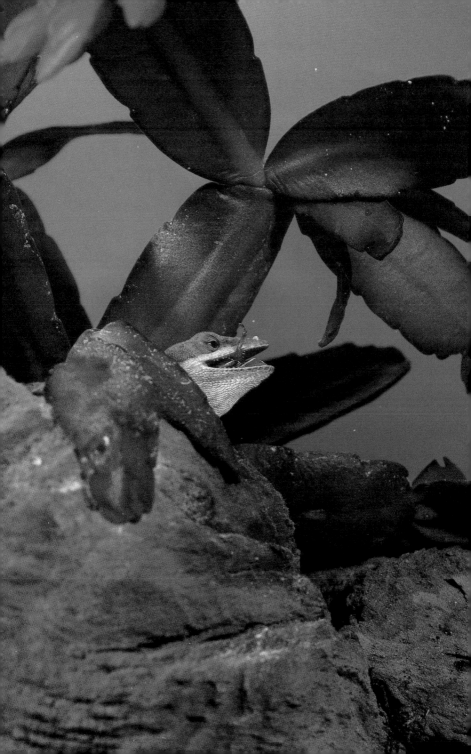

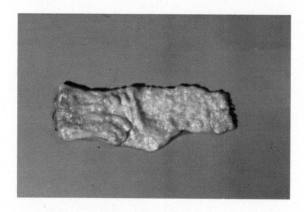

An inflammation of the gastro-intestinal mucosa can be recognized only after an autopsy. Here the intestinal walls are severely inflamed and the mucosa is a slimy, viscous mass.

Gastritis and Enteritis Gastritis is an inflammation of the stomach lining, while enteritis is a similar inflammation of the intestines. A gastro-intestinal disease often occurs parallel to an acute case of mouth rot and is probably caused by the stomatitis condition. Here we also find *Pseudomonas, Aeromonas*, and *Proteus* bacteria present. Progress of the disease ranges from simple inflammations of the gastric and intestinal mucous membranes (common gastritis and enteritis) to purulent abscesses and swellings or ulcerations.

Typical symptoms of a digestive tract disease are vomiting of half-digested food and soft, foul-smelling feces, nearly always accompanied by a purulent yellowish white mucus. Sometimes there are also traces of fresh blood. Often the pieces of inflamed mucous membranes are also excreted, frequently in

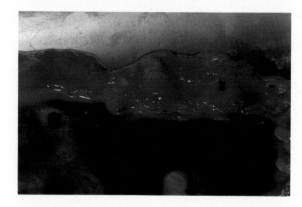

If an inflammation of the mucosa remains undetected for some time, it develops into acute purulent abscesses and tumors, which makes complete healing increasingly difficult.

conjunction with urine (the latter mainly in reptiles that spray urine as a defensive mechanism). The presence of pain and the discarding of the affected gastro-intestinal mucous membrane seem to play a more significant part, in conjunction with diarrhea.

If a cautious, gentle palpating of the digestive tract elicits a strong defensive reflex of the abdominal musculature (which tends to pull downward as a normal reflex), gastritis or

to the cotton swab are usually sufficient for a bacteriological examination.

Pneumonia Lung inflammations or pneumonia (in the broad sense) occur rather frequently in reptiles, usually as a consequence of other bacterial infections. The bacteria implicated belong—once again—to the *Pseudomonas* and *Aeromonas* groups; occasionally one can also differentiate *Mycobacterium* and

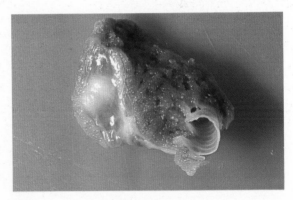

The possible formation of fibrin clots among the bronchial tubes or in the trachea represents a serious danger for reptiles that have colds or suffer from pneumonia. Such mucous and fibrin accumulations often lead to death by suffocation.

enteritis is indicated. In order to obtain material for bacterial examinations, the sick animal is gently massaged from the center of the abdomen toward the cloaca or a cotton swab is cautiously inserted into the cloaca. Stimulated by the massage, the animal usually gives off sufficient feces or mucous membrane, and the excrement fragments adhering

Pneumococcus. Similarly, lung inflammations are not too infrequently a consequence of mouth rot or bacterial gastro-intestinal disease. Yet pneumonia can also be the consequence of a sudden temperature drop, substantial cooling off, or a generally weakened physiological body condition.

The first symptom of

pneumonia is a whistling or rattling breathing sound made with a slightly open mouth, together with a nasal discharge, listlessness, and lack of appetite. During advanced stages there is a foamy and sometimes foul-smelling mucus given off from the mouth, together with very shallow breathing at a rapid frequency. In conjunction with pneumonia there is also the ever-present danger of fibrin clots developing and closing off large sections of the lung by blocking bronchial passages. This can ultimately lead to death by suffocation.

Treatment for pneumonia requires that the animal be kept in dry heat (about 30°C or 86°F). Apart from effective antibiotics (e.g., tetracycline treatment), eucalyptus vapor and a combination of vitamins A, B_{12}, and C, together with a mild circulatory medication (twice weekly, for two to three weeks) and infra-red light, have brought very good healing results. Heparin is injected in order to inhibit the formation of fibrin clots.

Tuberculosis Tuberculosis in reptiles is caused by

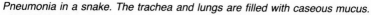

Pneumonia in a snake. The trachea and lungs are filled with caseous mucus.

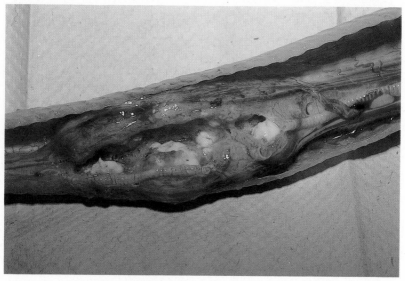

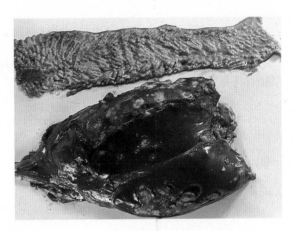

These organs, from a monitor that died of tuberculosis, were destroyed nearly beyond recognition. Reptilian tuberculosis is rarely diagnosed; if diagnosed, however, it rarely responds to treatment.

Mycobacterium. This disease is characterized by tumors and abscesses (nodules) on and in the skin, lungs, liver, and spleen, leading to destruction of the organ. Successful cures are extremely rare, so specimens with this disease should, for humane reasons, be euthanized.

Abscesses Abscesses are in essence encapsulated accumulations of pus, with a consistency ranging from watery-thin to cheesy-granular. Usually they occur as a consequence of secondary bacterial infections due to skin damage, feeding damage caused by ectoparasites (e.g., mites and ticks), as a result of housing that is too moist, or due to an inadequate or incorrect diet. Abscesses are

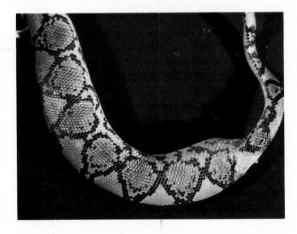

Plum-sized abscess caused by an injury. Well-developed inflammation in the cloacal region caused the skin and musculature to break. The abscess was successfully lanced and healed completely.

generally confined to the skin, but they can occasionally also inflict damage to internal organs. Abscesses in snakes are generally located under the skin. The affected organs in lizards are the skin, limbs, jaws with inner and outer lip margins, and a few other organs. In turtles the extremities are nearly always affected.

If an abscess is filled with watery-thin purulent matter it must be lanced and washed out with an antibiotic solution. Drainage should not be started in reptiles since these animals cannot be kept motionless. The wound should remain open under the dressing until healed from the inside out. The dressing should be changed once a day, the wound cleansed and then dressed again.

An abscess containing solid material can be cleaned out with a flat dental pick. Aggressive animals and those in which the abscess is on the jaw should be anesthetized because they would not keep still during the treatment. Lancing and cleaning out abscesses should be left to the veterinarian! Afterward, the wound is treated with antibiotic ointments or powders until it is completely closed.

Salmonellosis Reptiles— especially turtles—can continuously excrete *Salmonella* bacteria without ever being affected themselves by this disease. Cases of *Salmonella* poisoning so far diagnosed have nearly always originated in the country from which the animals (usually baby turtles) were imported. This organism is easily transmitted to other animals. Therefore, it is absolutely imperative that all newly imported reptiles be kept in quarantine for some weeks. During that period the animals should be closely checked for *Salmonella* by means of cloacal smears and fecal examination. *Salmonella* is all too frequently transmitted by means of insufficiently sterilized or disinfected equipment or other terrarium components and through the repeated offering of the same food organisms to different terrarium specimens.

Salmonellosis (actually a close relative of common food poisoning) is rarely recognized in reptiles (because there is a lack of clinical symptoms) until other negative influences take hold of the animal. Therefore, as a safeguard the feces should be

Opposite: Six-eyed pond turtle (Sacalia bealei), named for the two pairs of yellowish eye spots with dark centers usually found behind the eyes.

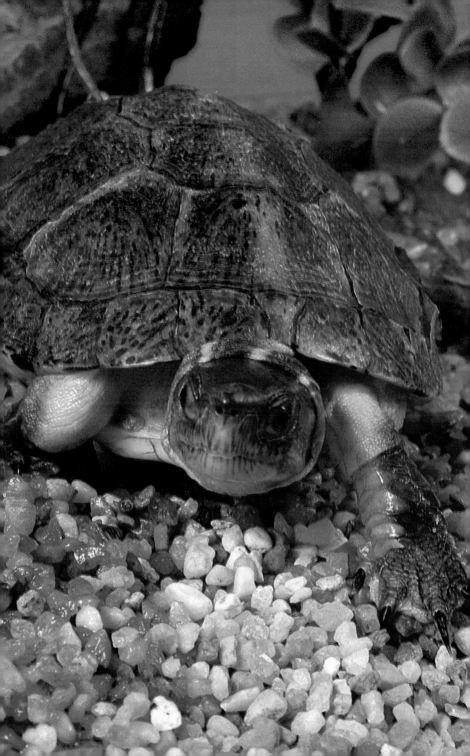

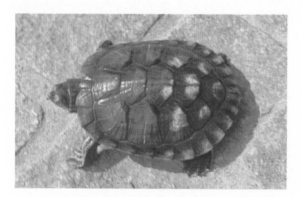

*Incorrect maintenance and care caused the development of fungi on the carapace of this red-eared slider (*Pseudemys scripta elegans*). Within a short period the fungus spread over the entire body and invaded the internal organs.*

examined regularly. If it has been shown that a particular animal is a *Salmonella* carrier, a six- to ten-day treatment with oxytetracycline has proven to be quite effective. In any case, after each contact with a reptile the hands *must* be disinfected properly. All small children must be kept far away from reptiles, especially young aquatic turtles.

FUNGAL DISEASES

Fungi live either on decaying plant and animal matter or parasitically on or in living plants and animals. They reproduce by means of branching (hyphae) or spores. Under suitably moist and warm conditions, fungi can spread very rapidly. Therefore, fungal diseases (mycoses) must be treated as quickly as possible.

It is not uncommon to find skin damage due to fungal attacks (dermomycosis) in reptiles, especially in those species that are kept in overly moist and warm terrariums. Usually the infection starts along the

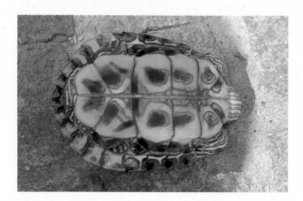

Underside of fungus-infected red-eared slider. The changes to the edges of the carapace are clearly visible and indicate a fungus infection.

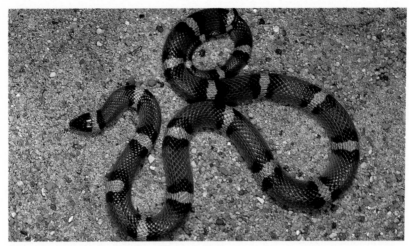

*A healthy milk snake (*Lampropeltis triangulum*).*

abdomen and manifests itself during the initial stage by raised brown-spotted scales. With a further spreading of the fungus large open, weeping wounds develop.

The most effective means of treatment of a mycosis is the identification of the specific fungus involved, followed by a specific application of a resistance-tested antifungal ointment or tincture. At an advanced stage of the disease this procedure, however, is too time-consuming and a trial-and-error method using different antifungals should be attempted in consultation with a veterinarian.

The sick animal should immediately be placed in a quarantine terrarium and maintained there under dry heat.

In the presence of open wounds, treatment is supplemented with antibiotics. So that they can dry out, the affected skin areas must *never* be covered. Before a completely cured animal is returned to its original terrarium, the entire container and its contents (decorations, etc.) must be meticulously disinfected and treated with antifungals. Fungal spores are extremely resistant and can lead—particularly among weak animals—to repeated new infections.

Fungal infections of internal organs can usually only be recognized at the advanced stage of this disease. In spite of so far largely unsatisfactory results, treatment should be attempted with an antimycotic (orally or injected i.m.).

Parasitic Diseases

DISEASES CAUSED BY PROTOZOANS

Unicellular organisms are microscopically small; they consist of only a single cell and reproduce by means of single or multiple division, budding, or through the fusion of nuclei. Many live parasitically in blood, in the digestive tract, and in other organs of animals. Under suitable conditions these organisms can cause considerable damage to the host and can even lead to its death.

Reptiles are hosts to numerous single-celled organisms in their blood and—mainly—in their digestive tract. Under normal conditions these parasites do not seriously affect the hosts or cause any damage. However, if a reptile is weakened for some reason (incorrect diet or care, stress, territorial fights, etc.) the parasites can suddenly reproduce uncontrollably and exert a considerable pathogenic effect.

Amoebiasis The most serious disease with the highest mortality rate is an infection with amoeba of the species *Entamoeba invadens*, which—due to its rapid epidemic-like progression—can wipe out an entire reptile collection. Under favorable circumstances (weak condition or small size of an affected host animal kept at a maintenance temperature of 18–25°C or 65–77°F) the infected animal can die within about two weeks.

Amoeba occur in two forms: an immobile, rather resistant permanent stage (cyst) and a motile, feeding, reproducing amoeboid stage (trophozoite). Reptiles take in amoeba as cysts via drinking water or food. The motile stage hatches from the cyst in the digestive tract of the host and there attacks and destroys the intestinal mucosa. The damage starts with an intestinal inflammation that in turn leads to small sores (ulcerations). Generally the intestinal tissue attempts to regenerate itself, so histological sections taken from an animal that has died of amoebiasis usually show a lamella-like layering at the affected intestinal segment. Prior to the discovery of these amoeba, this particular clinical picture (syndrome) was described as "membranous enteritis." With the disease advancing and the amoeba increasing rapidly in numbers, they penetrate actively into adjacent tissue or are transferred via the circulatory system into other organs, which

Opposite: The Asian wolf snake (Lycodon striatus) preys on lizards, such as geckos and skinks, and small snakes.

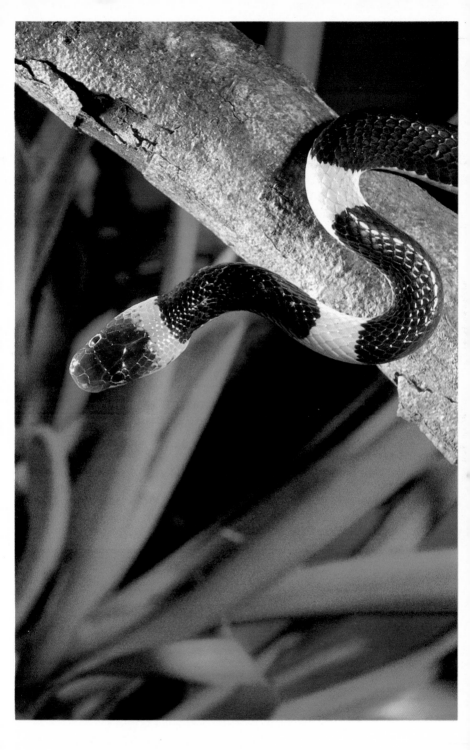

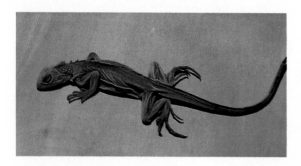

Poor results in treating amoebic diseases are due to late recognition. Once—or before—an animal looks this ill (caved-in musculature, etc.), a fecal sample should be taken for an immediate examination for amoebas.

can lead to serious liver and kidney damage.

The infected animals usually lie about lethargically, body extended on the ground. There is an increased liquid intake (lots of drinking). The coloration becomes pale and matte or often darkens. During further progress of the disease the animal regurgitates and generally food is refused thereafter. A purulent, slimy—even bloody—feces is a characteristic symptom of amoebiasis. At that stage there are severe ulcerative inflammations present in the digestive tract. This can lead to a hardening inside the last third of the tract that can be felt (under strong defensive reflexes of the abdominal musculature). The author also observed that the skin along the abdominal area can show reddish patches due to the inflammatory process. The presence of amoeba can be demonstrated in samples from slimy-bloody feces or smears taken from the rectum.

Treatment must commence as soon as any suspicion of amoebiasis is observed. The sooner treatment starts, the greater are the chances of recovery. The infected specimen should immediately be transferred to a quarantine terrarium. Tests have shown that raising the quarantine terrarium

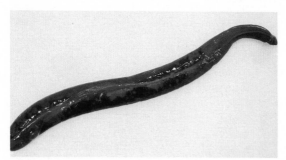

At an advanced stage of an amoeba infection, amoeba enter the blood stream and invade the liver and other organs, usually causing severe damage. In most cases, such a specimen can no longer be saved.

temperature to about 30–32°C or 86–90°F (not below 26°C or 79°F at night) tends to favor the healing process. When the temperature is increased it is imperative that the animal always has sufficient fresh drinking water available. An effective medication for amoebiasis is, for instance,

disease has been eliminated. Almost any effective treatment for amoebiasis should be done or directed by a veterinarian.

Although the reptilian pathogen *Entamoeba invadens* bears considerable resemblance to the human pathogen *Entamoeba histolytica*, it does not appear to have any

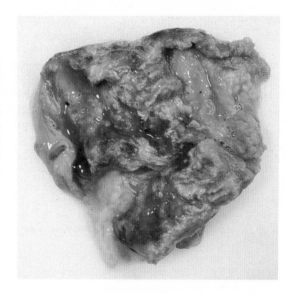

Changes in this intestine were caused by a Trichomonas *infection. Hemorrhaging areas indicate where the intestine became fused, thus inhibiting the passage of food.*

metronidazole. It is administered orally for up to one week at 25 mg/kg body weight.
Suppositories inserted into the cloaca as well as additional antibiotic supplements support the treatment. About four weeks later another smear should be taken to determine whether the

detrimental effect on humans. Nevertheless, great caution and painstaking hygiene must always prevail when handling sick reptiles!

Trichomondas Other single-celled organisms that are not uncommon in the intestine of reptiles and cause a similar clinical picture as *E. amoeba* are flagellates of the genus *Trichomonas*. Newly imported reptiles especially seem to bring trichomonads with them.

Slimy, purulent feces and a general deterioration of the animal's overall condition—although not to such an extent as in the case of amoebiasis—is characteristic of a *Trichomonas* infection. Histological sections taken from dead specimens show necrotic, purulent, or tumor-like changes of the digestive tract and stomach; smears and histological sections indicate a massive infestation with trichomonads.

Metronidazole has proven to be quite effective against *Trichomonas* infections.

WORM DISEASES

Worms are elongated, usually bilaterally symmetrical invertebrate animals. Many of them live parasitically in animals. Representatives of flukes (Trematoda), tapeworms (Cestoda), nematodes (Nematoda), and spiny-headed worms (Acanthocephala) and their larval stages occur as parasites or pathogens in reptiles. Many of these worms undergo several larval stages during their development, which in turn involve different hosts. Since the life cycles of most of these worms are rather complicated, a detailed description is omitted in this book. Instead, we will deal with only the pathogenic characteristics, the identification

*Left: Massive nematode infestation in the gastro-intestinal tract not only forms a blockage but also causes widespread tissue damage. **Right**: Nematodes occur not only in the digestive tract; some species invade the lung and can cause death by suffocation.*

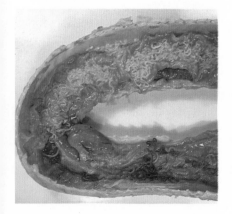 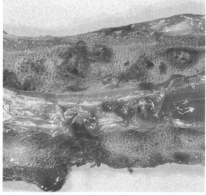

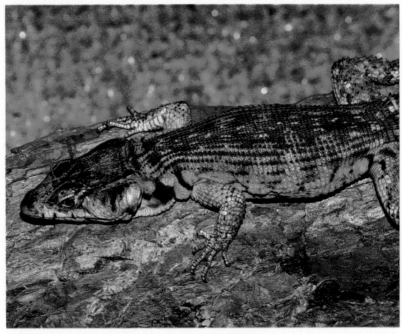

*A false girdled lizard (*Pseudocordylus microlepidotus*).*

of some groups of worms, and their eradication.

In·order to implement a specific medical treatment, you must know what worms have infested a particular animal. This can easily be determined by the examination of a feces sample, which—if there is indeed a worm infestation—always contains a number of eggs that give an indication of the group of worms involved. Since prevention is always better than a cure, any responsible reptile keeper should have feces samples from all of his charges examined regularly. For that purpose a small piece of fresh feces is placed in a well-sealed plastic tube that is sent off to the nearest veterinary laboratory. This tube should be clearly marked with the name of the

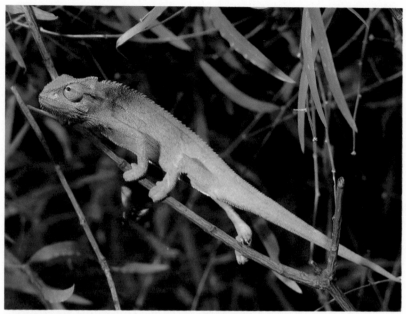

*Double-banded chameleon (*Chamaeleo bitaeniatus*)*.

reptile species concerned. Mixed or "mass" fecal samples are regrettably too often sent out for examination, but these are essentially useless since they may well give a positive or negative result but without identifying the specific animal(s) that are actually infested with worms.

Nematodes (Nematoda)
Among those worms that parasitize reptiles, nematodes take the top rank. These worms invade nearly all organs but seem to prefer the stomach and intestinal tract and the lungs, primarily in carnivorous and carrion-feeding species. Heavily infested reptiles show—in spite of their food intake—a mounting loss of condition, apathetic behavior, loss of coloration (paling), and sometimes also diarrhea, caved-in musculature, and sunken eyes.

Autopsies of dead animals usually indicate massive infestations of the digestive tract by nematodes that often have invaded the abdominal cavity, resulting in large purulent inflammations with abscesses along the stomach and intestinal walls, encapsulated cysts on or in the organs, or peritonitis. The latter is invariably due to the fact that intestinal fluid entered the abdominal cavity through holes in the intestinal wall. Stomach- and intestine-invading nematodes include mainly members of the Ascarida, Oxyura, and Strongylida.

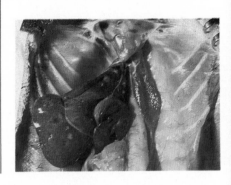

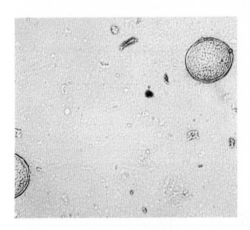

Above: Larval forms of nematodes can cause severe damage to the host as in this decimated liver. **Left:** Ascarid eggs (250X). **Below:** Hatching of an ascarid larvae from an egg.

Ascarid eggs are round with a thick shell; oxyurid eggs are oval, flattened on one side, and contain (in part) embryos; strongylid eggs are elongated, rounded off, with a thin shell, and also contain more or less well-developed embryos.

When recognized at an early stage from regular fecal examinations, nematode infestations can be effectively eradicated by treating with

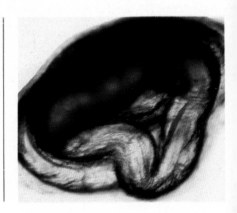

piperazine and tetramisole compounds. Late identification and/or delayed treatment inevitably leads to massive infestations that usually are fatal.

Far more difficult to deal with are nematodes invading the lung (rhabdites), the circulatory and lymphatic vessels (filaria), and nematodes that settle in tissue (dracunculids). The presence of these in a host is difficult to detect, and they are regrettably only noticed on the basis of extensive damage to the host, such as blockages of circulatory or lymphatic vessels, necrosis, edemas, skin sores, abscesses, and pneumonia.

If a filaria infestation is suspected, it is recommended that you take blood smears without delay. If these are positive, a treatment with diethylcarbamazine can

sometimes produce a cure in mild cases.

Tapeworms (Cestoda)
Tapeworms (Cestoda) can invade the digestive tract of reptiles as sexually mature worms or as eggs. In the event of massive infestations or when already weakened animals are attacked, this can cause extensive damage to the host since these worms tend to place a severe drain on its nutrition. Cestodes can also lead to inflammations of the intestinal mucosa and to intestinal blockages.

Adult tapeworms can live inside a reptilian host for years without causing any externally visible detrimental effect on the host. Yet, with regular fecal examinations cestodes can easily be detected, either

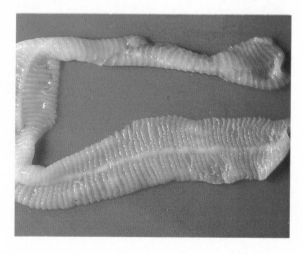

Tapeworms are not uncommon in reptiles. Eggs and segments from adults can easily be seen in fecal samples.

Right: Tapeworms regularly shed segments filled with eggs, thereby assuring perpetuation of the species. *Below:* Tapeworm taken from an anaconda (Eunectes *sp.*).

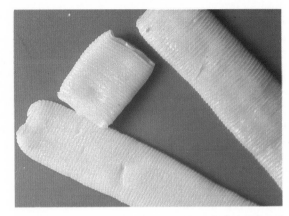

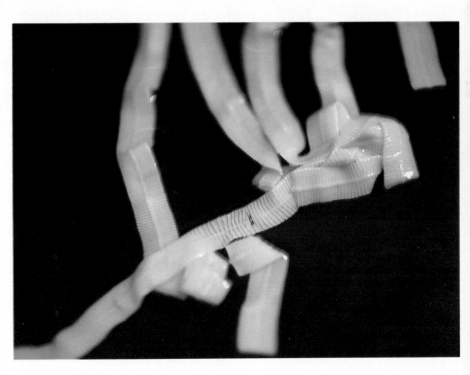

through the presence of their eggs (round and thick-shelled eggs with three pairs of hooks clearly visible on the embryo) or on the basis of shed yellowish white flat body segments (proglottids). Even when the affected animal does not display any adverse symptoms, tapeworms should be eradicated. A single oral administration of niclosamide,

migrations inside the host's body and cause substantial damage to organs and tissue. Regrettably, such damage usually can be detected only during autopsies of dead animals, since the external clinical picture does not give any indication of larval cestode infestation. Severe damage to the liver and musculature usually causes death.

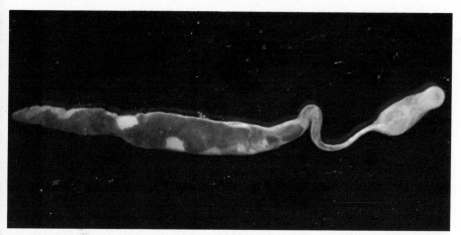

*A trematode or fluke (*Macrodera longicollis, *a common pulmonary parasite of snakes) taken from a grass snake (*Natrix natrix*).*

bunamide, or methyl benzene (carefully following dosages prescribed by your vet) usually is sufficient to accomplish this. On the other hand, cestode larvae are much more pathogenic, since they undertake extensive

Flukes (Trematoda) Flukes (trematodes) can occur in reptiles in the urinary and gall bladders, digestive tract, kidneys, liver, lungs, and circulatory system. Although this group of worms is not

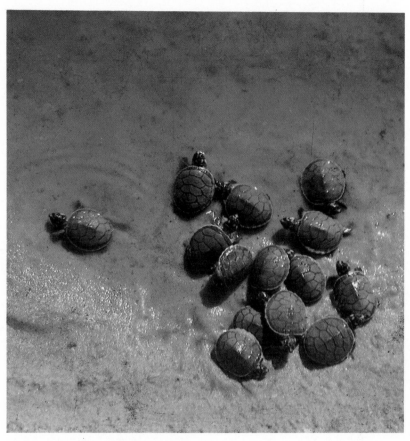

*A group of yellow-spotted Amazon turtle hatchlings (*Podocnemis unifilis*). Newly imported turtles occasionally carry leeches.*

particularly rare (trematode eggs can be found in the feces and urine), pathogenic symptoms on a large scale are not known to occur in reptiles. Apart from that, specific treatment for the

eradication of these worms is rather difficult.

Leeches (Hirudinea)
Occasionally newly imported turtles and crocodiles carry

leeches. Apart from their blood-sucking activity and the possibility of abscess formation, they do not adversely affect their host. Whether diseases are transferred by leeches has not yet been investigated. Leeches can easily be removed by dabbing some alcohol onto them and then pulling them off. The bite sites should be treated with antibiotic ointment or powder in order to prevent an infection through bacteria and other organisms. They normally heal completely in a short period of time.

MITES AND TICKS

Mites are relatively small (0.1 to 7 mm), spider-like animals with a compact, unsegmented body bearing four pairs of legs (during the larval stage only three pairs) and with biting or sucking mouthparts. Numerous mite species live parasitically on or in animals and man, where they can cause considerable damage to the host.

Reptiles are attacked primarily by "blood mites" (*Ophionyssus*) that settle mainly in the axillae of the limbs, at the base of the tail, around the eyes, on the abdomen, and underneath the scales. They can act directly as damage-causing parasites (blood sucking, skin damage) and also can transmit many other pathogens (filaria, bacteria). These tiny reddish brown organisms can under favorable moist and warm conditions reproduce in vast numbers in a few short weeks. Massive infestation, if in young reptiles or those under stress, can cause the host's death.

If reptiles are seen rubbing or scratching along rocks and branches and if they seem to enter their bathing container unusually frequently (especially if the water surface is subsequently covered with many tiny dark dots), these are signs of a mite infestation.

There are various methods to eradicate these parasites. The

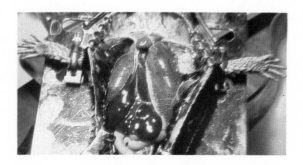

Parasitizing mites and ticks not only inflict damage by constantly sucking blood from the host, but the bitten areas also permit secondary infections. Moreover, mites and ticks can also transmit various disease germs directly into the host.

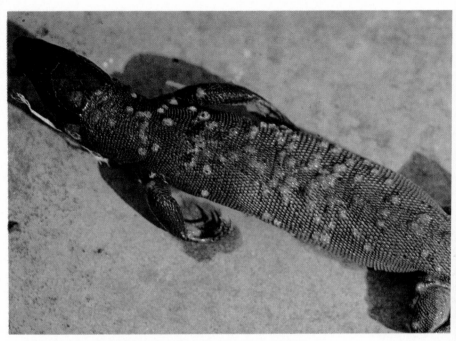

*Green or emerald lizard (*Lacerta viridis*) infested with ticks.*

affected animal can be rubbed with cod liver ointment and then placed inside a white cotton sack (to be changed daily) until finally mites can no longer be found on the animal and inside the sack. Alternatively, the cotton sack can be sprayed with a 0.2% solution of trichlorfon; once the sack is completely dry the animal is placed inside for about 12 hours. *Never* apply the spray directly to the affected animal! Caution must be exercised with juvenile animals placed inside such pretreated sacks—there may occasionally be slight cases of poisoning!

The author has often achieved better and more rapid results with propoxur sprays and powders: the head of the animal is covered and the body is sprayed (against the scales) from a distance of about 15 cm. The eyes, lips, and head regions are cautiously dabbed with a cotton swab previously sprayed with propoxur. The animal is then placed inside the cotton sack. After a short period of time the mites start to fall off. Treatment must be repeated until the last mites have hatched from eggs under the scales and are subsequently also eradicated. At the same time the entire terrarium and its contents must be emptied out and disinfected. This procedure must be thorough and has to be repeated. Substrate and branches should not be reused since they may be infested with mite eggs that will start up another mass infestation. Once all mites have been eradicated it is advisable to place the animal in a luke-warm camomile bath before returning it to a now clean and well-ventilated terrarium.

Many hobbyists have used a desiccant powder to control mites, with variable results. Follow the manufacturer's instructions carefully. Currently many prefer to put a piece (about thumb-nail size) of pesticide-impregnated plastic strip (sold under many brand names) at the top of the cage for a two- to three-day interval every few weeks. Both methods work well and are relatively safe with larger reptile specimens.

Treatment of inflammed bite areas should be done with an antibiotic ointment, which always produces quick healing. Vitamin supplements given with the normal diet further improve the overall condition of the animal.

Ticks are slightly larger than most mites (actually, they are very large mites themselves) and occur in reptiles only as ectoparasites. They exert a detrimental influence on the host by sucking substantial amounts of blood and/or transmitting blood filaria. In most cases they can easily be removed with the aid of a pair of blunt forceps. Ticks should be picked off by cautiously turning them briefly left and right before pulling them out. It is important that the mouthparts be extracted to reduce the chance of infections. If a tick is too firmly attached, cover it with petroleum jelly so the parasite suffocates and then simply drops off. Bite wounds should be treated with antibiotic ointments.

Opposite: Galapagos marine iguana (Amblyrhynchus cristatus). *This species is now considered endangered; in addition, it has long been considered inappropriate for the terrarium. Time, effort, and money will be spared if you take the time to choose the right species for your resources. Careful planning will be beneficial to both you and your future reptilian pet.*

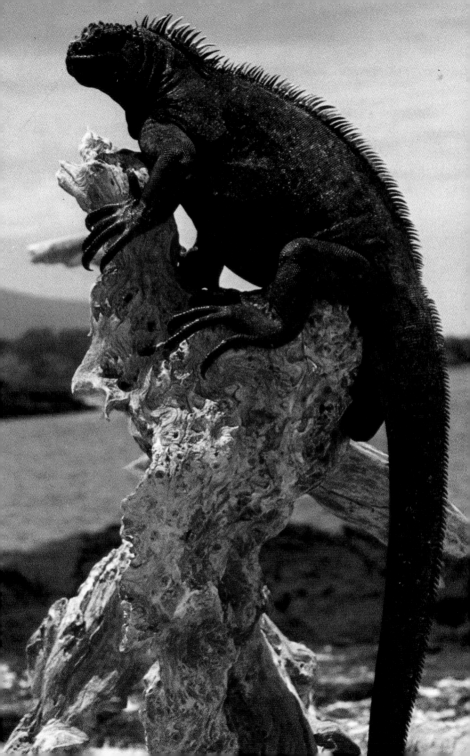

Environmental Diseases

Among environmentally induced diseases, those due to poor or incorrect maintenance and/or inadequate nutrition are the most significant. This is particularly regrettable since there is sufficient relevant literature and there are also many clubs and associations dedicated to the maintenance, nutrition, and breeding of reptiles!

OVER-FEEDING

Reptiles in captivity are more likely to die due to obesity than starvation. On one hand this is due to a vastly one-sided diet and on the other because the animals are being fed far too often. Are there really still hobbyists who make the modest effort necessary to collect meadow plankton (small insects) for small lizards? Who still maintain in their homes or apartments various food breeding colonies such as waxmoth larvae, fruitflies, and crickets? Who collect earthworms and snails for their turtles, geckos, or snakes in order to provide some variation to the diet of their charges?

A highly varied diet not only protects against obesity due to a monotonous commercially available mealworm diet, but it also persuades many reptiles that are refusing to feed to resume normal feeding. There are, however, food specialists among reptiles, such as horned lizards (*Phrynosoma*) that feed only on ants, snakes that will feed only on lizards, and even snakes that feed mostly on their own smaller siblings. For these animals the best advice is: let them find their own food—in their native habitat; you are doing yourself and the animal concerned the greatest of favors by leaving it alone.

The food requirements of a particular reptile specimen are dependent upon its size, age, environmental temperature, and activity. For instance, many snakes can do without food for quite some time, and therefore in captivity they (at least the larger species) should really only be fed at most every two weeks. The author is aware of many cases where snakes have refused food for more than ten months, remained perfectly healthy, and then finally resumed feeding. If feedings are too frequent or if too much food is offered at one time, the food is not properly utilized and the excess is stored as fat. Geckos, for instance, maintain fat reserves in their tails for "hard times." If these surpluses become too large they

*Opposite: A mandarin rat snake (*Elaphe mandarinus*). This species feeds mainly on small mammals, killing prey by constriction.*

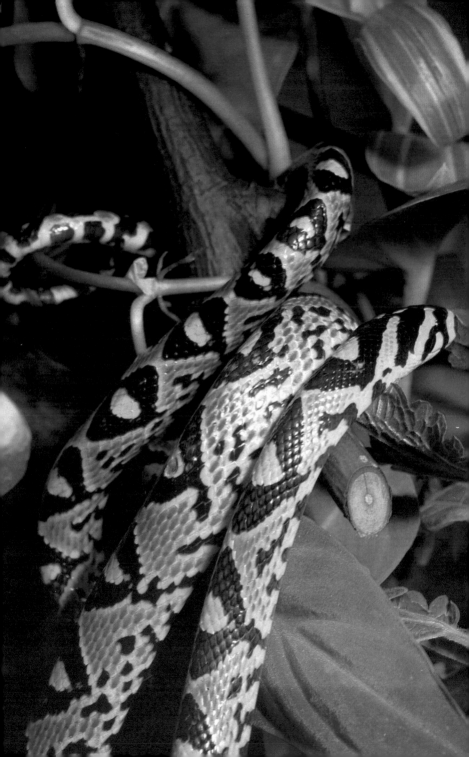

are stored not only at the intended reserve sites, but also around or in internal organs, so that these are eventually no longer fully functional.

Degeneration of the liver, cardiac and arterial inclusions due to calcium deposits (sclerosis), calcification of the kidneys and their ducts, formation of kidney and gall stones, whitish yellow urea deposits in the liver and kidneys, and arterial sclerosis due to cholesterol and calcium deposits (sometimes resulting in complete blockages) are often consequences of too much food. If these conditions have already advanced too far and organs have become affected on a large scale, a reversal (and cure) is hardly ever possible.
Unfortunately, recognition of such conditions is often rather difficult. Therefore, it is advisable to maintain some fasting days for the animals as a preventive measure.

VITAMIN DEFICIENCY (AVITAMINOSIS)

Vitamins are absolutely essential nutritional substances that often cannot be produced (or are produced in insufficient quantities) by most animals and which therefore have to be taken in via the food. (A few vitamins are synthetized in the body of various species and thus do not have to be present in the food.) A one-sided or incorrect diet will quite often lead to serious vitamin deficiency diseases (avitaminosis). For instance, vitamin D deficiency causes the softening of bones, rachitis, and

Due to overfeeding, these internal organs, especially the liver, show crystalline deposits which seriously impaired normal functioning.

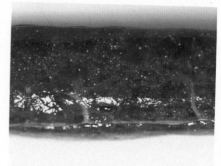
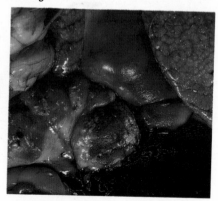

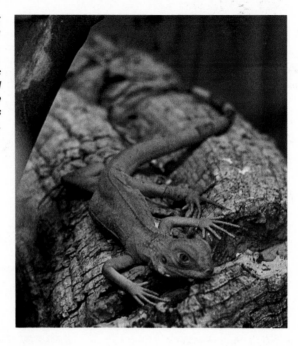

Vitamin deficiency manifests itself in abnormal growth, softening of bone, crippling, and apathetic and disinterested behavior. This little lizard needs vitamins urgently.

loss of teeth, and facilitates bone fractures, carapace softening or deformation in turtles, and white spots on the carapace of painted turtles. Vitamin A deficiency leads to eye damage such as clouding and swellings and to skin infections. Vitamin B deficiency in lizards leads to paralytic symptoms in the hind legs and at the base of the tail and to acute digestive disturbances. Molting and growth problems, mouth rot, skin changes such as spots, cracks, and loss of coloration (paling), and increased lack of resistance to infections can all have their origin in an acute vitamin deficiency.

Treating avitaminosis involves considerably more than just offering sufficient vitamins with the food. It is somewhat simpler with herbivorous reptiles than with carnivorous ones. For the former there are numerous fruits and vegetables available. Honey, a few crumbs of yeast, small pieces of heart, liver, and muscle meat, waxmoth larvae, or one- or two-day-old mice supplement the (ideal) varied diet. The more diverse the diet, the greater is the benefit to the animal. In order to find out what exactly is eaten by a particular species and specimen it is best to use the trial and error method.

Carnivorous reptiles should be given food animals or pieces of meat impregnated with multivitamin preparations. Some carnivorous reptiles also like to feed occasionally on fruits and sweet vegetables that have been coated with vitamins. A carnivorous reptile diet can be further diversified by adding some wheat bran, oatmeal, egg yolk, plant seeds, and finely chopped up fish. Specimens that take only live foods should get their vitamins via the drinking water, or the food animals can be injected with the necessary vitamins just before they are offered to the reptiles.

In their early stages vitamin deficiency diseases can still be corrected relatively easily through proper dosages of vitamins given over a prolonged period of time. However, changes in bone structure, eye clouding, carapace deformations, and similar damage cannot be corrected. Vitamin D deficiencies such as softening of bones and rachitis should be treated with precisely dosaged vitamin D and calcium supplements as well as with additional UV radiation. *Caution:* excessively prolonged UV radiation is harmful! Do not place the UV lamps closer than 80 cm from the animal. The exposure time must not be longer than three minutes. UV radiation treatments given just twice a week are perfectly adequate.

VITAMIN EXCESS (HYPERVITAMINOSIS)

Anyone under the impression that pumping reptiles full of vitamins is doing his animals a favor is totally wrong! Vitamin

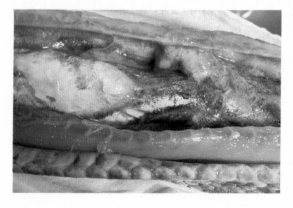

Left: *Too many vitamins can be fatal! Here, excess calcium and vitamin supplements had a detrimental effect on the heart and aortic arches and normal circulation could not be maintained.*
Opposite: *Pancake tortoise (*Malacochersus tornieri).

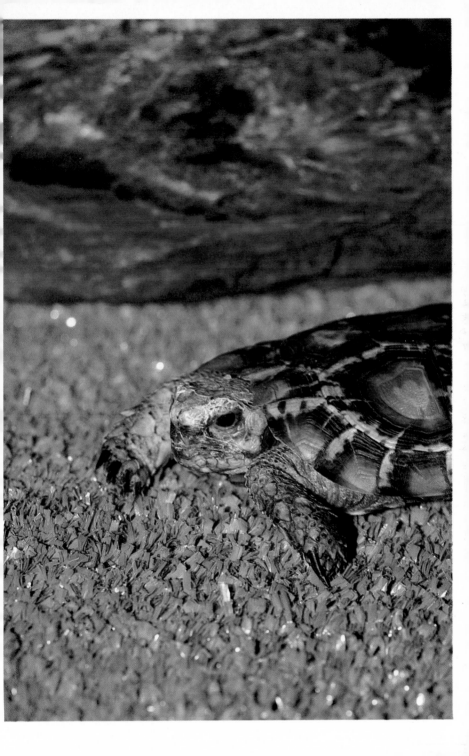

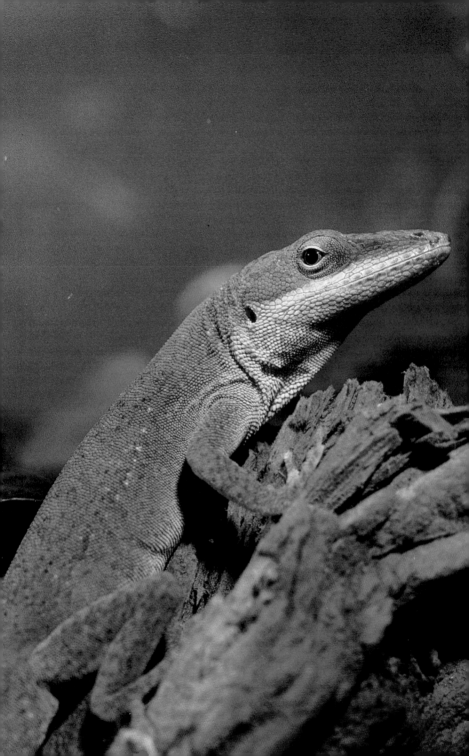

dosages that are consistently too high can sometimes lead to damage as serious as that caused by not enough vitamins. For instance, excessive vitamin D supplements can cause the onset of calcification of the arteries, and uncontrollable bone and cartilage growth can occur. Too much vitamin A can lead to uncontrollable bleeding in the internal organs. The author has encountered such vitamin excess diseases (hypervitaminosis) mainly in juvenile specimens that had been given well-intentioned but excessive vitamin supplements.

CALCIUM

Calcium carbonate (limestone) and other calcium preparations are not—as is often erroneously assumed—vitamins, a point that is to be stressed. Regrettably, hobbyists often administer (as a "preventive measure") calcium carbonate as tablets or in other forms. Reptiles excrete excess salts mainly via the kidneys and Harder's gland. If, however, there is an excess of calcium it is deposited in the form of calcium accumulations in kidney tissue, along heart walls and arteries, and sometimes also in the musculature and the bones. Occasionally kidney and gall stones are formed that usually cannot be removed without surgical procedures.

Therefore, juvenile specimens should only be given a small amount of calcium in the form of crushed egg shell or cuttlefish bone or via Ringer's solution

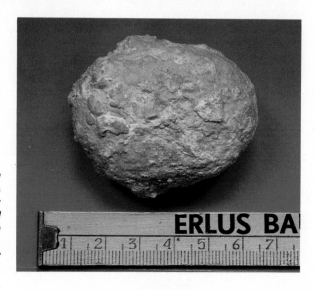

*Opposite: A green anole (Anolis carolinensis). **Right:** Overfeeding and additional calcium supplements produced this kidney stone.*

every three months. Additional calcium supplements are not required when a well-balanced, varied diet is given. The skeletons of food animals (vertebrates and invertebrates) always contain sufficient calcium.

EDEMAS

In certain snake species and in desert-dwelling geckos the

COLDS

Colds are not too infrequently the consequence of inadequate care—drafts, cold bathing water, excessive temperature variations, and high humidity can all play a significant role when reptiles show signs of nasal discharge, weeping eyes, coughing, and sneezing!

During the early stages colds can be treated effectively with

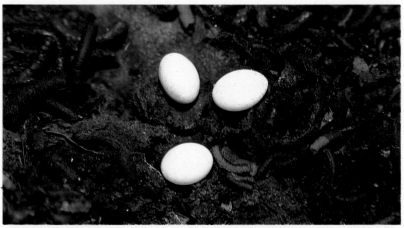

A trio of Anolis *eggs. Calcium is necessary for proper egg production, but too much can be very dangerous.*

author has observed the formation of edemas (swellings due to the accumulation of a fluid in tissue gaps) in the skin and axillae of the limbs that were probably due to the fact that the animals had been kept too moist. Pathogens could not be found in the fluid.

heat and infra-red radiation and by massaging the chest and nasal region of the affected animals with eucalyptus oil. Modest vitamin C, A, and B_{12} supplements may expedite the healing process. Advanced stages of colds must be treated with antibiotics without delay.

DIGESTIVE PROBLEMS

An incorrect diet can sometimes lead to diarrhea and similar gastric disturbances. These problems can quite often be cured with medical carbon tablets added to the food or alternatively with pieces of banana and apple, which are animal incapable of finding its own food, so it has to rely solely on the keeper. It may, however, be more humane to put the animal down.

INTESTINAL PROLAPSE

Diarrhea as well as constipation in reptiles can

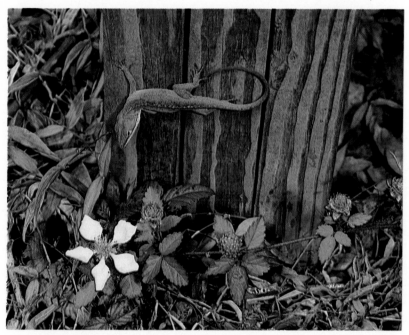

Green anole (Anolis carolinensis*). Most digestive problems can be avoided by feeding a species-correct diet to your reptile.*

eagerly eaten by nearly all lizards and turtles.

Injuries to the tongue and the upper jaw where the taste and olfactory organ (Jacobson's organ) is located render the cause a prolapse of the rectum, whereby a more or less large section of the rectum protrudes from the cloaca. As long as there is no tissue damage such a prolapse can be moved back into

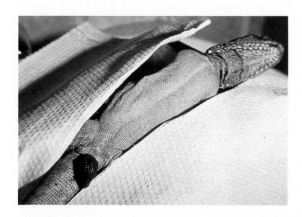

The intestinal prolapse of this lizard was treated with the help of a physiological saline solution; subsequently, it was put back into the proper position.

place by a veterinarian. It is important, however, to place a wet bandage cautiously around the cloacal region as soon as this problem is noticed. This prevents the protruding section of the intestinal tract from drying out and facilitates the reformation of the intestinal mucosa. If a prolapse is not promptly discovered and the protruding section has already turned dark blue to black, only a quick surgical removal of the protruding section will prevent even more serious injury. Such an operation can easily be done on an otherwise healthy reptile and usually leads to quick recovery.

EGG-BINDING

Poor maintenance conditions, stress, the activity of other terrarium occupants, and lack of suitable egg-laying sites can all be causes of egg-binding in female reptiles. Unfortunately, egg-binding often is diagnosed only during an autopsy. If a female shows signs of a swelling in the cloacal region or a cloacal prolapse, you should—in the absence of other obvious causes—suspect a case of egg-binding. If this happens only a surgical procedure will save the animal.

MOLTING PROBLEMS

A varied diet, species-correct care, and adequate bathing facilities are the best preventive measures against molting problems. Even then it can happen that a particular specimen molts only badly or incompletely. An incomplete molting can give rise to various skin diseases, such as scale rot (necrotic dermatitis).

Molting difficulties can be corrected with warm baths and by massaging cod liver oil onto the affected areas. Do not remove the remaining skin fragments by force, because this can lead to inflammation. Be particularly careful around the eye area—leave it to an experienced veterinarian. You can make his task easier by applying petroleum jelly to the affected eye before you take the animal to a veterinarian. Similar results also can be obtained by touching up the eye area with a cotton swab soaked in warm water.

INJURIES DUE TO INCOMPATIBILITIES

Injuries among reptiles due to placing together incompatible species or specimens are not rare. It does not take much to imagine what would happen if a snake that feeds on lizards were

Female bull snake (Pituophis melanoleucus) expelling an egg. Egg-binding is dangerous and often deadly; the hobbyist should strive to prevent rather than treat this condition.

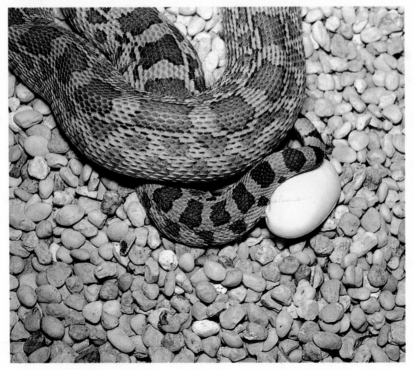

placed together with such potential prey. An experienced hobbyist would not be surprised if under such circumstances the lizards would seem to "disappear."

from the way they do in the wild, particularly when the space is limited. Well-defined territorial behavior and insufficient flight space often lead to serious fights. Additionally, competing

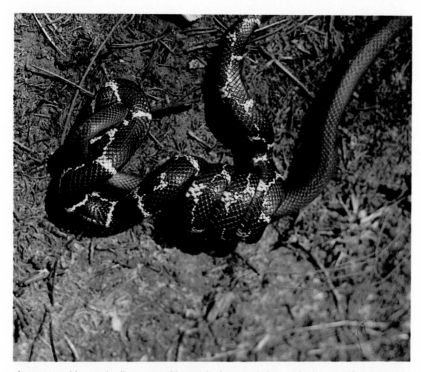

An eastern kingsnake (Lampropeltis getulus) *constricting a black racer* (Coluber constrictor). *Before housing numerous reptiles together, be sure they are compatible and that one won't prey upon another.*

When several reptiles are placed together into the same terrarium the animals should initially be closely monitored. Even sibling specimens in captivity behave totally different

for food, never-ending dominance fights among males over females, and excessive activity occur in an over-crowded terrarium or when incompatible species are kept together in the

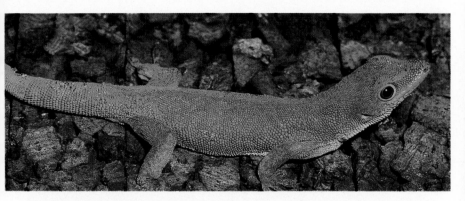

If a terrarium is occupied by several animals, there is always the possibility of aggression, often resulting in injuries or loss of limbs.

same terrarium. The outcome of such intense aggression may include bitten-off tails and toes and even mortalities. Animals exposed to such stress are easy targets for various infections. Moreover, give some thought to a pregnant female that has to find a suitable place to deposit her eggs in such turmoil!

ACCIDENTS

Carelessness, ignorance, and lack of true concern by the

*Eastern hog-nosed snake (*Heterodon platyrhinos*) eating a toad.*

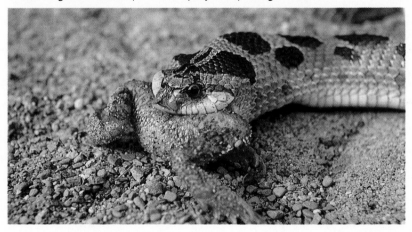

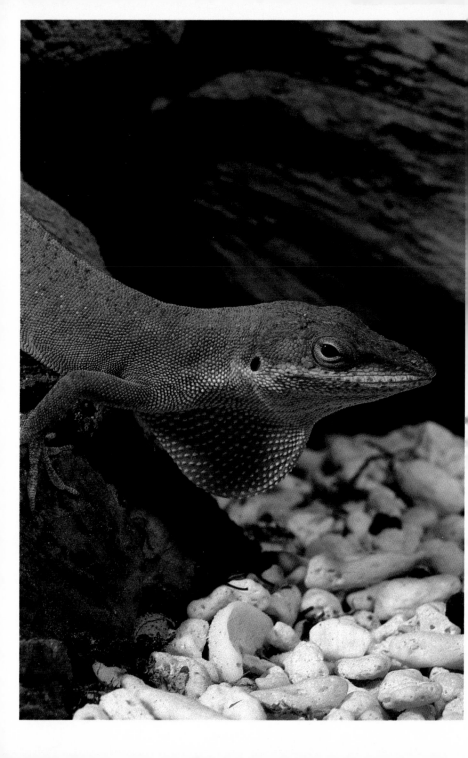

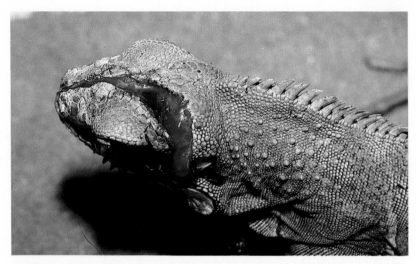

Opposite: *Green anole (*Anolis carolinensis*).* ***Above:*** *A female iguana (*Iguana iguana*) that was injured by an aggressive male. This bite penetrated the bones of the skull.*

hobbyist can easily lead to injuries that could be avoided. One reasonably common occurrence is that reptiles become wedged among or are even killed by inadequately secured rock structures or branches in the terrarium. Unprotected lamps and heaters or those that are placed too low or otherwise incorrectly placed inside the terrarium often lead to serious burns. Sharp rocks and branches, protruding points of screws and nails, cracked drinking water containers, and the wrong "tools" can cause cuts. Careless, rough handling inside the terrarium can cause abrasions and fractures.

Incorrect application of medication, disinfectants, insecticides, and herbicides, as well as insufficient washing of fruits and vegetables or dandelions and clover picked by the side of the road, is known to have poisoned many reptiles. Bathing containers that are too deep without providing proper climbing stones have led to many drowning deaths among captive reptiles.

Terrarium doors that do not close properly and lizard tails hanging out of a terrarium are welcome toys for cats. While such accidents may sound strange indeed, these and many more that seem even more

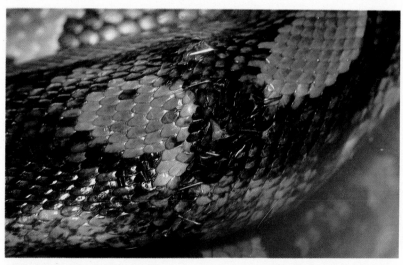

Reticulated python (Python reticulatus) with a severe laceration caused by a fight with a cagemate. The laceration is held together with metal sutures.

bizarre have really happened!

Ruptures, stings, cuts, and bites must be treated with an antiseptic powder or ointment. When protected by antibiotics most of these wounds heal without further complications. Larger and deeper wounds should be treated—if need be surgically—by a veterinarian. During the subsequent molt these areas should be closely monitored since there may be minor problems over healed wounds. Additional support may have to be provided in the form of warm baths or ointments.

Torn or bitten tails are usually regenerated (autotomy) by lizards. Some reptiles even regenerate lost toes. Slight superficial burns are treated with 1% tannin or cod liver ointment.

In case of suspected fractures manifested by dragging or hanging of the affected extremities or through abnormal positions, the animal should be x-rayed and the fracture properly attended to by a veterinarian. The fracture is secured with a firm bandage and checked after about four weeks. This is sufficient time for the complete healing of fractures. Substantial swellings may occur in conjunction with fractures; these should be treated with anti-inflammatory ointments.

Inflammations due to minor bruising can also be treated with anti-inflammatory ointments. If after severe bruising reptiles show paralysis, if they bleed from the mouth or nose, or if the animal does not recover within a short period of time, it should be euthanized in order to avoid unnecessary suffering.

If a tail or even a leg is badly bruised or otherwise injured and complete healing can no longer be expected, it is recommended—in order to avoid general septicemia—that that extremity be amputated. The animal will no longer look flawless, but even if missing a limb it is only marginally incapacitated in its mobility and can still give much pleasure to the hobbyist.

POISONING

Poisoning in reptiles—due to feeding of lettuce leaves, fruits, and vegetables that have been sprayed with chemicals, food organisms that have come into contact with insecticides, and poisonous fumes (e.g., disinfectant remnants)—manifests itself in apathy, vomiting, and diarrhea. Severe poisoning symptoms include serious cramps, convulsions, and respiratory problems. In such cases rapidly provided first aid is of paramount importance! Unregurgitated food (should this be a problem) should be brought up by inducing the animal to vomit. Bathing in water at 30 to

Green anole (Anolis carolinensis). *Keep in mind that many plants are poisonous for reptiles.*

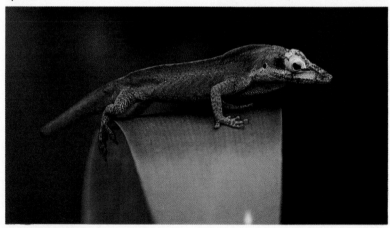

33°C (86–92°F) contributes to emptying the digestive tract. If bathing does not work, a mild but rapidly acting laxative is administered. Mild metabolic medication prevents a collapse of the circulatory system and supports the animal's overall constitution. In cases of

This blue-tailed day gecko (Phelsuma cepediana) lost part of its tail during a territorial fight. Unfortunately it did not grow back properly.

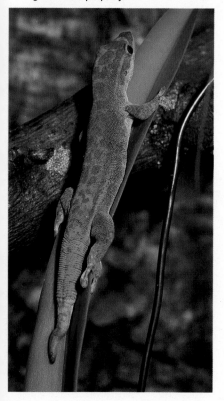

poisoning due to noxious fumes or an insufficiently ventilated, freshly disinfected terrarium, the affected animal should immediately be transferred and well-ventilated. *Caution:* drafts must be avoided!

TUMORS

Since research into the formation of tumors—be these benign or malignant, real tumors or mere swellings—in reptiles is still in its infancy, a detailed description of the different types is omitted here. Moreover, in most cases a cure can not be expected. Tumors can occur anywhere in and on the body; no organ is immune. They grow more or less rapidly and are essentially unpredictable. Depending upon their location, size, rate of growth, and onset of metastasis, they mean in nearly all cases an eventual death of the affected animal. Only in cases of benign tumors can—depending upon location and size—an early surgical removal save the animal. In all cases this would require an experienced veterinary surgeon. As long as the affected animal is not suffering and does not have to be kept alive by force-feeding and there are no other problems, such an animal can still be kept. In all other cases euthanasia is the preferred option. Whether such tumors can be transferred from one animal to another and

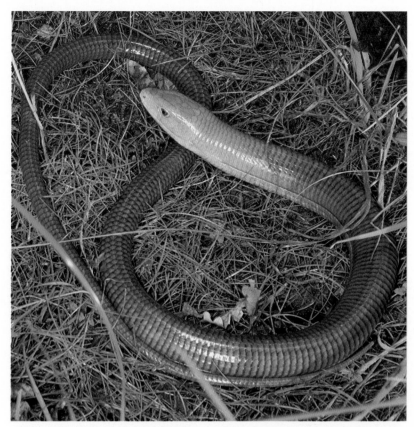

*Glass lizards, like the sheltopusik (*Ophisaurus apodus*), are called "legless" because, except for rudimentary hind legs in some species, limbs are primarily absent.*

whether food organisms play a part in tumor formation have not yet been resolved.

ANOMALIES

Anomalies such as abnormal skin coloration and double or multiple heads, tails, or limbs should remain untreated as long as they do not have a detrimental effect on the animal. In those cases where the normal life of an animal is severely restricted and there is no realistic medical solution, euthanasia is recommended. Prolonging the life of reptiles with serious physical afflictions is indeed cruel—in the wild such animals would not survive for long.

Some Reptile Psychology

In comparison to a life in the wild, the environmental conditions of reptiles in captivity vary substantially—however, their innate type of behavior remains unchanged. In order to be able to provide adequate species-correct housing, a good reptile keeper must also know something about the psyche of his charges as expressed in their movements and changes in shape and coloration. He must be informed about the territorial and courtship behavior, the warning and display behavior, mock fights and submissive gestures, the avoidance of enemies, and the search for food. Such knowledge can be acquired through reading the relevant literature and through discussions with other reptile hobbyists, but primarily through constant and precise observations of one's own animals.

Therefore, the terrarium should be set up in such a way that if it is occupied by several animals (of either the same or different species), each animal has adequate space and sufficient cover (hiding places) and flight possibilities in order to escape from the attacks of stronger opponents. Animals that actively search for food must have enough space to move about. On the other hand, animals that gather food more passively must find sufficient camouflage and cover. Diurnal animals must be fed during the day or under artificial illumination, while crepuscular and nocturnal species prefer dusk and darkness.

If the animals are closely and frequently observed their behavior often indicates what is required and what is missing. For instance, in a smaller terrarium weaker animals are constantly exposed to mock fights, such as territorial fights, that usually have detrimental effects on them. Decisive for well-defined territorial behavior are, however, not only size, age, and strength of an animal, but also the time spent in a particular terrarium. Therefore, it is not advisable to place newly arrived specimens into a well-established terrarium that already contains well-established specimens. The new arrivals—often weakened and under stress from shipping and change of habitat—are never able to stand up against the display and territorial behavior of the established animals. Instead they will have to surrender with submissive behavior, which

Opposite: False map turtle Graptemys pseudogeographica). Before setting up a community terrarium, be sure that all species have proper temperature and humidity, ample hiding and egg-laying places, and other environmental essentials.

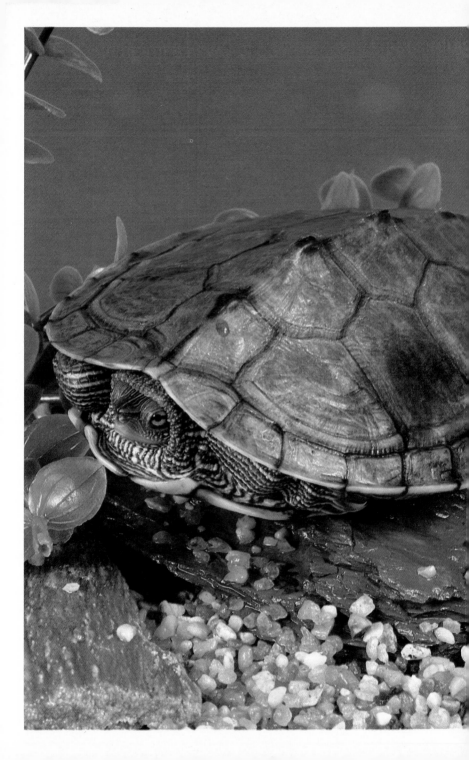

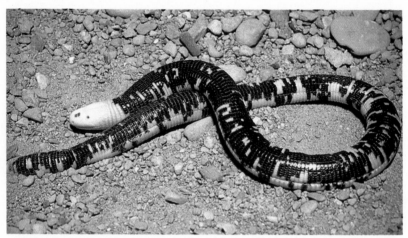

*Speckled worm lizard (*Amphisbaena fulginosa*). Worm lizards are primarily predators, but will often accept dead food in a proper terrarium.*

possibly can even lead to their death.

Submissive behavior is particularly easy to observe in lizards; however, it must not be mistaken for similarly exhibited courtship behavior. Submissive behavior usually manifests itself by either placing the body flat on the ground together with closed eyes, or through rapid "stomping" with the forelegs. This type of behavior usually stops the attack of the stronger opponent prematurely. If this behavior is seen among animals of the same sex, they should be separated or transferred into a larger terrarium with more hiding places.

Have you ever closely observed your animals when they are in pursuit of prey and noticed how the tail twitches in excitement before they attempt to charge their intended prey? In reptiles, the tail is a particularly important means of expression of moods. For instance, the tail may be used to fend off an attacker (the typical rattling in rattlesnakes), to indicate excitement (in many lizards by twitching motions), or in order to court a female. Yet there are still many other possibilities to demonstrate display, threat, or courtship gestures. These include, for instance, the spreading of often colorful skin flaps on the throat (the dewlap or gular pouch) together with opening of the mouth in a threatening gesture (*Anolis,* agamids, certain other lizards), changes of coloration (chameleons), rhythmic movements of the head and body, and loud hissing (snakes). Such intimidation tactics express extreme alertness and are intended to signify that such a warning must not be ignored, otherwise there will be a fight.

These means of expression can be arranged into three categories that should be observed, particularly by those hobbyists who keep aggressive or venomous species. This categorization is appropriate since reptiles indicate quite clearly and unmistakably—not only to their own kind but also toward humans—how far their

"intimate sphere" can and may be invaded. In snakes a slight hissing or "spitting," a moderate spreading of the throat sac in lizards, and signs of imminent fleeing in lizards and turtles indicate a first stage warning. If at this point the animals are left unmolested these signs will subside rapidly and the animals return to their normal behavior. If, however, these warnings are not heeded, the hissing and "spitting" become more intense together with a nervous twitching of the tail. Lizards at this second stage will display their dewlaps more strongly, take on their so-called "shock coloration," erect themselves to appear larger in most of the

The brown anole (Anolis sagrei*) spreads its dewlap during courtship and in territorial disputes.*

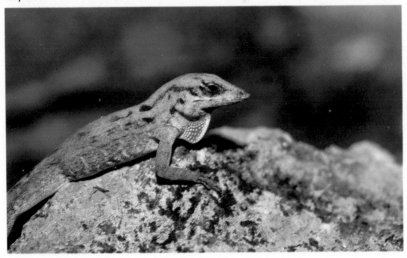

large lizards (agamids, monitors, etc.), and keep their tails in a ready-to-whip position. Turtles at that stage will retract into their carapace. If at that stage the animals are left in peace again, they will remain in their respective defensive positions, watching closely and critically their immediate surroundings.

The third stage represents extreme alarm readiness, clearly indicating that the animal is now taking things quite seriously. Now the disturbed animal moves into a serious defense readiness position or will even attack. Snakes tend to coil up with the head retracted like a steel spring into the middle of the coil. Nervous, rapid tongue-flicking facilitates quick orientation toward the opponent; striking with an open mouth indicates a direct attack. This is followed by actual bites (venomous snakes will then give off venom). Lizards during the third stage will try to whip their opponents with the tail and they will also use their strong jaws in bite attacks, sometimes securing firm bites

*Boa constrictor (*Boa constrictor*). When preparing for an attack or defense, most snakes coil up and prepare to strike.*

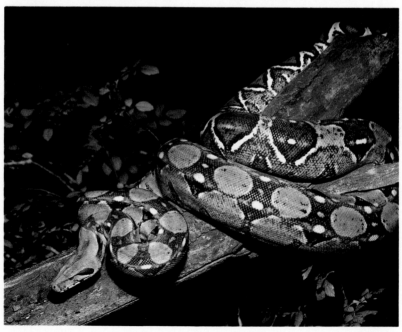

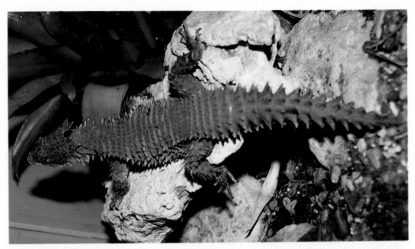

*Sun-gazer (*Cordylus giganteus*). During the stage of alarm readiness, many lizards prepare to whip opponents with their tails.*

on the opponent. Foul-smelling secretions are now given off (either sprayed or simply excreted). Turtles hide inside their carapace, and many may try to bite their opponents from that position.

It is amazing to see the energy and persistence used by sometimes even small reptiles in order to defend themselves, even when the opponent is much larger and stronger. If all this is in vain, some reptiles will then use deceptive techniques that represent a clever passive defense, such as faking death, forming a ball, turning sharp spines and thorns toward the outside, or even dropping their tail in order to confuse an enemy.

Intraspecific display, threat, and courtship behavior proceed slightly differently and according to well-defined rules that are usually adhered to closely. Close monitoring and constant observation will quickly show what the substantial differences are. It would be a totally mistaken belief now to say that territorial fights can be eliminated by keeping the animals in individual housing. This would indeed be quite wrong, because social interactions with all their display and submissive behavioral forms are essential for the animals to reach and maintain their normal activity. In a well laid-out and suitably decorated terrarium containing branches, plants, rocks and rocky structures, several watering sites, and heat and light sources, a normal social order among all resident reptiles can develop without constant rivalry fights.

Reptiles have vastly differing individual characters: some are placid and shy, others are aggressive and ready to bite.

become "hand tame" (but they can not be trained to perform). So-called "panic merchants" are sometimes difficult to deal with, though. These animals will—as soon as they see someone approaching—go into a real panic and attempt to flee. They have a tendency to run into the glass sides, causing bruised and

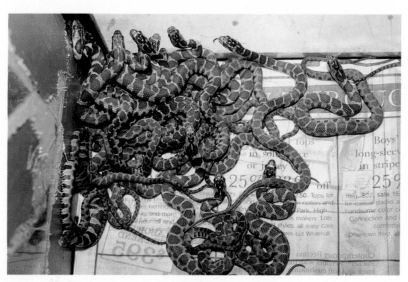

*A litter of young common water snakes (*Nerodia sipedon*). No animal likes to live in overcrowded conditions. Keep this in mind when setting up your terrarium.*

There are rarely ever problems with the quieter species. They will in time become used to the keeper and will take food from the keeper's hand. Lizards, particularly, have a tendency to

bleeding heads and mouths. For these animals the terrarium should be set up in such a manner that branches, rock structures, and plants extend all the way to the front glass so that they can find a suitable hiding place quickly. Under such conditions the animals settle down more easily and tend to lose some of their shyness. This, however, does not mean that some of the terrarium's interior

need be when the keeper approaches will in most cases try to flee first before they bite. If there are sufficient hiding places for such animals, there is then rarely any need for the animals to attack.

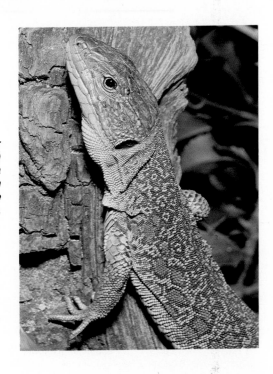

*The ocellated, jeweled, or eyed lizard (*Lacerta lepida*) should be kept in a moderately damp terrarium with climbing branches; the temperature should be stable.*

decoration can be taken out again once the animals have "calmed down"; most lizards, especially basilisks, will quickly fall back into their old panicky behavior patterns.

Other specimens that do not exhibit any fear and may even use their strong teeth and jaws if

Reptiles that like to bathe and also use water as an escape route are also quite common. For these animals a small, shallow water dish would be inadequate, since they need a large water bowl. Experiences in captivity have shown that animals that need water to

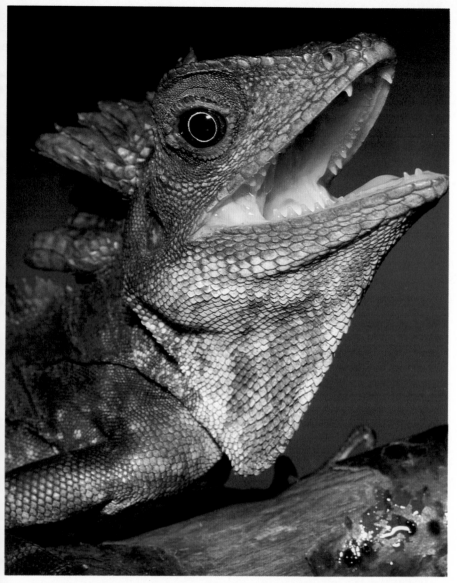

Agamid lizards open the mouth in a threatening gesture during courtship and fights.

escape into but were not given this opportunity did not feed properly and displayed molting difficulties. A small episode observed by the author will illustrate this point. A water bowl for an aquatic agamid had been emptied for a few days for reconstruction. A visitor wanted to have a closer look at the animal. Since the animal felt threatened, it jumped from its resting place on a branch directly into the empty basin, closed its eyes, and rowed with body and tail as if there were water in the basin. After a short period the animal raised its body and viewed its surroundings. Since the "intruder" was still close by, the animal "dove" and again closed its eyes and continued to "swim" along. As cute as this incident may seem, it clearly demonstrates the strength of innate behavior.

Another unusual type of behavior unrelated to molting or any other influence was observed in various lizards. These animals jumped into water, turned and shook their body, and then scratched with their front and hind legs any place that could be reached on their body. These baths took a long time and were executed quite meticulously. Afterward the animals were so exhausted that they withdrew to their resting site close to a heat source, where they let their extremities hang down and slept until dusk. They were then briefly active again, and finally retired for the night. This behavior gave the impression of a regular grooming session. In order to avoid health problems the water temperature must never be higher than the ambient air temperature, otherwise the animals are likely to catch a cold when they come out of the water. It is recommended that the water temperature be kept between 18 and 20°C (65–68°F).

Medications for Sick Reptiles

Sick reptiles are a problem for every reptile fancier, particularly so since there are few veterinarians who are specialists. There are, however, a number of medications that have proven to be effective in the treatment of reptile diseases. Some of these are available only with prescriptions, while others can be purchased only from pharmacies. It is of paramount importance to seek expert advice from a veterinarian, an experienced reptile hobbyist, or a zoo before any animal is given medication, since an incorrect treatment can do more harm than good.

The following tables list proven (tested) medications for the treatment of bacterial and fungal diseases; for the eradication of single-celled organisms, worms, mites, and ticks; for the treatment of colds, gastro-intestinal diseases, burns, bites, bruises, and vitamin deficiencies; and for the disinfection of wounds. Many of the drug brand names listed are also available as generic drugs that are equally effective. Your veterinarian will know what equivalent drug to prescribe.

Below: This sheltopusik (Ophisaurus apodus) was the victim of an improperly installed heating device. Note how well the burn healed with proper treatment. Opposite: Malayan snail-eating turtle (Malayemys subtrijuga).

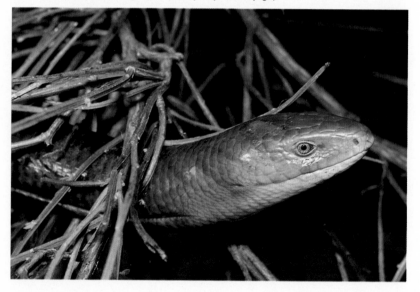

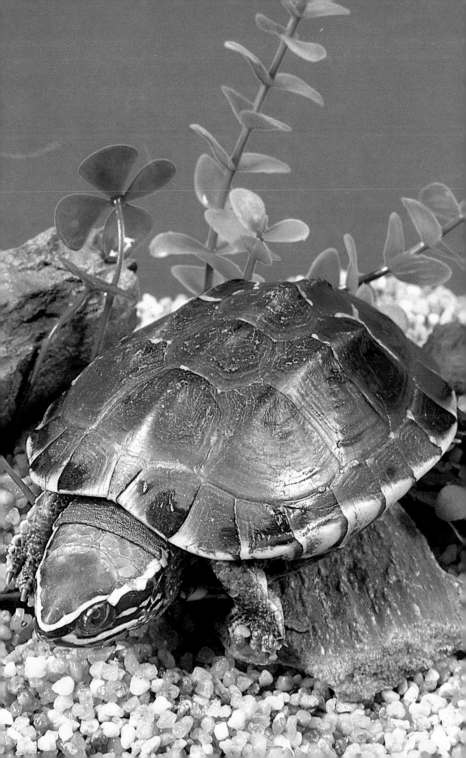

MEDICATIONS FOR SICK REPTILES

BACTERIAL DISEASES

Medication (act. ingr.)	mg/ml/kg body wt.	Applic.	Frequency	Diseases	Remarks
Aureomycin	30-50 mg	i.m./i.p.	1× daily 3-4 days	mouth rot, pneumonia, diseases of g.i. tract	increased dosage for smaller animals
Bisolvon	3 mg	i.m.	1× daily	pneumonia	also give 0.1 ml/kg Heparin to prevent formation of fibrin clots in bronchia
Chloromycin	50-60 mg 15-30 mg	orally orally	1× daily 1× daily	g. i. tract diseases, pneumonia, large purulent abscesses	1st day high dosage, from 2nd day low dosage
Chloramphenicol spray		extern.	2-3× daily as needed	abscesses after lancing, eczemas, purulent wounds	until wound has healed
Fucidine Gauze with 2% ointment		extern.	1× daily	external bacterial wounds and abscesses	cover with dressing until healed
Gentamycin	10-15 mg	i.m.	1× daily	mouth rot and g.i. tract infections, bacterial infections	toxic to kidneys; not to be used for prolonged periods
Hexoral spray		extern.	2× daily	inflammation of oral mucosa and onset of mouth rot	
Nebacitin eye ointment, Scherisona F eye ointment		extern.	1× daily	bacterial eye diseases and infections	until completely healed
Nebacitin powder, ointment cones		extern.	1× daily	purulent wounds & abscesses, bites, eczemas	until completely healed; cone size dependent upon size of wound
Supronal supens. 20%	0.5-1 ml	orally, rectally	1× daily 4-7 days	mouth rot, g.i. tract	to be painted on after wound has been cleaned; several times for mouth rot
Supronal	0.5 ml	i.m.	1× daily 2-3 days	mouth rot, bacterial infection	give in drinking water for small animals, 0.1 ml/100 ml
Terramycin, Tetracyclin	40-60 mg	i.m./i.p.	1× daily 3-5 days	nearly all bacterial infections	lower dosages for new arrivals; supplement with vitamin A and C inject. for mouth rot

NOTE: Juvenile specimens should be given lower dosages, adult specimens higher dosages.

Opposite: *A pair of green anoles (Anolis carolinensis). Green anoles are known for their love of warmth.*

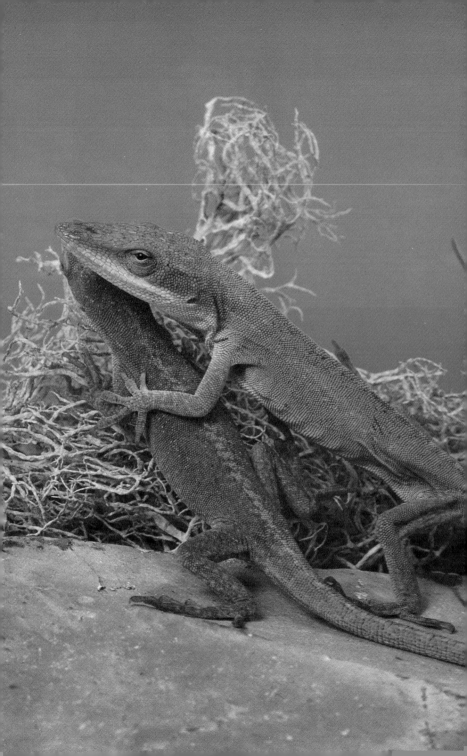

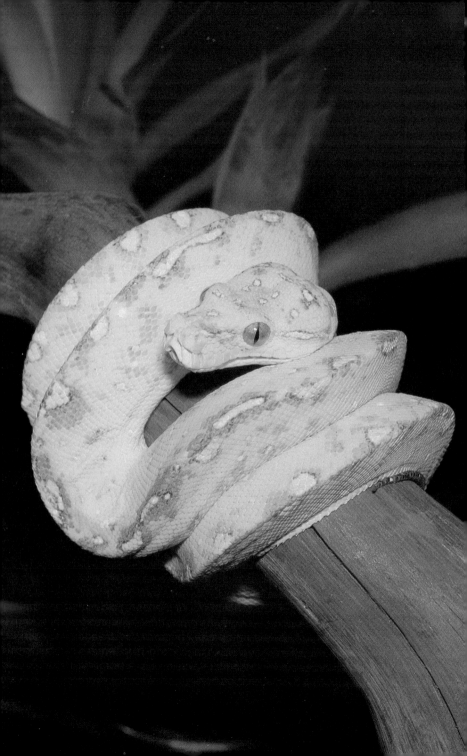

FUNGAL DISEASES

Medication (act. ingr.)	mg/ml/kg body wt.	Application	Frequency	Remarks
Daktar i.v.	1.5 ml	i.p.	1 × daily every 2 days, 4-5 times	use when internal fungus infection is suspected
Daktar i.v.	5 ml per liter	external	1 × daily bath for 15 min.	for turtles, etc., per 1 liter bathing water for large infection
Daktar ointment, powder		external	1 × daily	treatment until completely cured, rub in or powder and keep dry; fungus infection of skin
PHISO hex		external	2 × daily 2-3 minutes	external fungus diseases, applied locally; let it take effect for some time and then rinse off with clear water; keep animals dry. Treatment until cured.

PROTOZOAN DISEASES

Medication (act. ingr.)	mg/ml/kg body wt.	Application	Frequency	Remarks
CLONT (tablets)	30-40 mg	orally	1 × daily 6-8 days	dissolve tablets in water; for enteritis use 35 mg/kg body weight. Simultaneous injection of Ampicillin. Give lots of liquid
CLONT (suppositories)	30-40 mg	cloacally	1 × daily 2 days	
Resochin	1 ml	i.p.	1 × daily 6-8 days	also for amoebiasis; simultaneous administration of antibiotics (e.g., Terramycin). Possible side effect: vomiting has been observed

MITE AND TICK INFESTATIONS

Alugan		extern.	1 × daily	0.3% solution for washing animals, do not rinse off; continue until all mites have disappeared; if needed repeat in 2 weeks.
Bolvo Spray		extern.	1 × daily	spray *against* scales; protect head, dab around eyes with cotton swab; purulent abscesses to be treated with antibiotic ointments.

Opposite: *A young green tree python (*Chondropython viridis*). Tree pythons incubate their eggs on the ground; brooding animals should be protected from all disturbances.*

MEDICATIONS FOR SICK REPTILES

WORM INFESTATIONS

Medication (act. ingr.)	mg/ml/kg body wt.	Application	Frequency	Diseases or Condition	Remarks
Citarin Sln 10%	0.5 ml	i.p.	1 ×	nematodes	
Droncit	5 mg	orally	1 ×	tapeworms	increases dosage 5-fold for *Bothridium*; may need to be repeated
Fenbendazol	40-60 mg	orally	1 × daily 2 days	nematodes, oxyurids, ascarids, and others of g.i. tract	administer with some water; can also be given in food
Helmex	15 mg	orally	1 × daily	ascarids, hookworms, oxyurids	for 3 consecutive days in case of serious hookworm infestation
Mebendazol	80-100 mg	orally	1 × daily	for nearly all Nematoda	3-5 days, depending on infestation
Panacur	40-50 mg	orally	1 × daily	Nematoda of g.i. tract	not effective for all nematodes (oxyurids, ascarids)
Resochin	25-40 mg	orally	1 × daily 2 days	Trematoda	
Telmin KH	100 mg	orally	1 × daily	ascarids	possibly repeat when positive
Thiabendazol	40-60 mg	orally	1 × daily 2 days	ascarids, oxyurids, Trematoda	single dose repeated after 14 days

Opposite: A green anole (Anolis carolinensis) *in the process of swallowing an insect.*

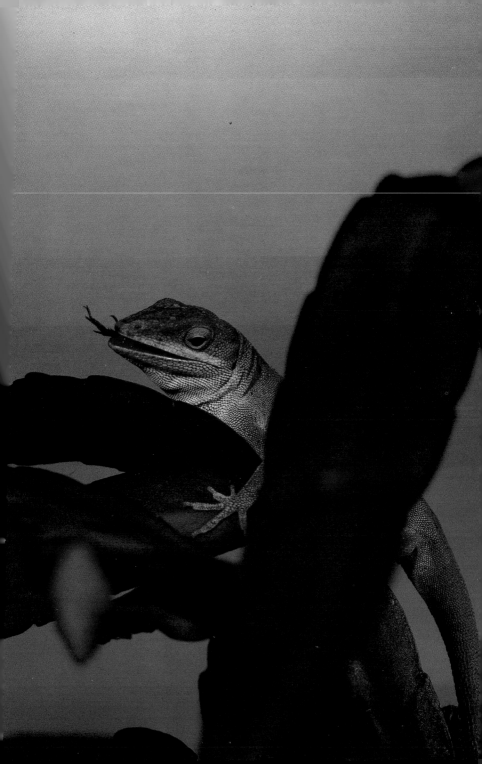

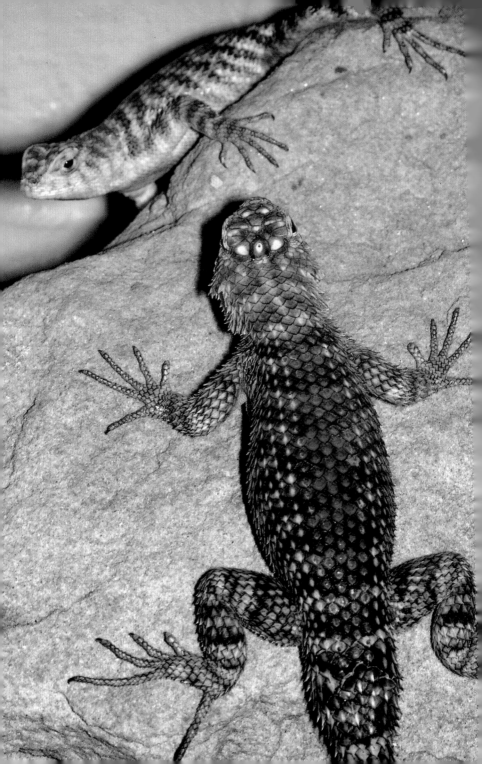

OTHER DISEASES

Medication (act. ingr.)	mg/ml/kg body wt.	Application	Frequency	Diseases	Remarks
Kamillosan	refer to manufacturer instructions	oral & external	1 × daily	colds	to be inhaled, 5 drops/50 ml lukewarm water
				constipation, g.i. tract diseases	
				cloacal abscesses & inflammation	administer baths until healed
				pharyngeal and jaw injuries	painted on until healed
				molting difficulty around eyes	use strongly diluted
Kamillosan Ointment		external	1 × daily	open bite wounds, scratches, injuries to extremities	treat until healed
Scheroson F		external	2 × daily	1st degree burns, eczemas, inflammations with closed fractures	
Tannalbin tablets	¼ tablet	orally	1-2 × daily	diarrhea	decrease food
Terramycin Spray		external	1-3 × daily	small open wounds and burns	
Vitamin Paste 100		orally	1 × weekly 4 weeks	vitamin deficiencies, prevention of vitamin deficiency diseases	about pea-size drops together with food, after 4 weeks stop for 3 months
Kodan Spray		external	1-2 × daily	Wound disinfection	disinfection agent
Mirfusot Bath		external	1 × daily	diseases of respiratory tract	to be inhaled, 10 ml/1 liter lukewarm water
Nuran BC forte	2 ml	orally	1 × week 4 weeks	vitamin deficiencies	pea-size drops given with food; after 4 weeks stop for 3 months.
Osspulvit		orally	2 × week	softening of bone and carapace	app. ¼ tspn given with food; after 2 weeks stop for 2 months.

Opposite: *A pair of desert spiny lizards (*Sceloporus magister*); female in background, male in foreground. According to some experts, desert spiny lizards need temperatures above 37°C (98°F) for proper digestion.*

Suggested Reading

THE COMPLETELY ILLUSTRATED ATLAS OF REPTILES AND AMPHIBIANS FOR THE TERRARIUM
By Fritz Jurgen Obst, Dr. Klaus Richter, and Dr. Udo Jacob
ISBN 0-86622-958-2
TFH H-1102

Here is a truly comprehensive and beautiful volume covering all reptiles and amphibians any hobbyist (or scientist) is likely to ever see or want to know about. The alphabetical arrangement makes it easy to find information on almost any topic, and the more than 1500 full-color photos make this book a pleasure to look at as well.

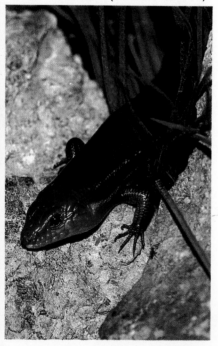

Blue-tailed skink (Eumeces fasciatus).

ENCYCLOPEDIA OF REPTILES AND AMPHIBIANS
By John F. Breen
ISBN 0-87666-220-3
TFH H-935

This book provides enormous coverage of the care, collection, and identification of reptiles and amphibians. Broken down by animal type, it is written for either the amateur or professional herpetologist, making it of value to anyone interested in herptiles.

BREEDING TERRARIUM ANIMALS
By Elke Zimmermann
ISBN 0-86622-182-4
TFH H-1078

This volume covers everything the hobbyist needs to know about the successful breeding and rearing of terrarium animals, including housing, terrarium, light and heat, breeding food animals, and many other essential topics. In addition to the superlatively informative text, this book contains over 200 full-color and black and white photos.

Index

Abscesses, 65
Accidents, 99
Amoebiasis, 70
Anomalies, 105
Autopsy, 50
Bacterial infections, 52
—medication chart
Bathing dish, 24
Calcium, 93
Cleanliness, 25
Colds, 94
Defensive "rigor," 9
Diet, 16   *pg 20 -22*
Digestive problems, 95
Disease, recognition of, 38
Display behavior, 108–115
Drinking containers, 24
Edema, 94
Egg-binding, 96
Enteritis, 62
Fasting period, 16, 18
Flukes, 80
Fungal diseases, 68
—medication chart, 121
Gastritis, 62
Housing, species-correct, 16
Incompatibility, 97
Intestinal prolapse, 95
Leeches, 81
Lizard anatomy, 34
Medication, administering, 45

Mites, 82
—medication chart, 121
Molting problems, 96
Mouth rot, 54–60
Nematodes, 76
Over-feeding, 86
Pneumonia, 63
Poisoning, 29, 103 *(40)*
Protozoan diseases, 70
—medication chart, 121
Quarantine
—period, 13
—temperature, 43
—terrarium, 14
Salmonellosis, 66
Signs of health and illness, 10, 40
Snake anatomy, 32
Submissive behavior, 106, 108
Tapeworms, 78
Ticks, 84
—medication chart, 121
Trichomonads, 73
Tuberculosis, 64
Tumors, 105
Turtle anatomy, 36
Viral infections, 52
Vitamin deficiency, 88
Vitamin excess, 90
Worm diseases, 74
—medication chart, 122

Vomiting   pg 40

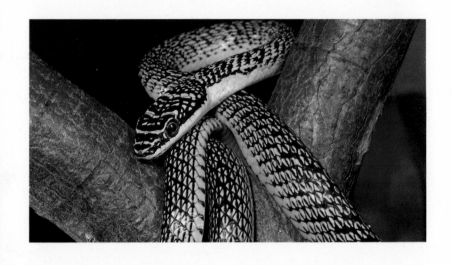

REPTILE DISEASES
KW-197